Contents

Introduction

Healthy Eating is Volume 408 in the **issues** series. The aim of the series is to offer current, diverse information about important issues in our world, from a UK perspective.

About Healthy Eating

A healthy diet is essential to our overall wellbeing but it is not always possible to achieve. Research has shown that healthy foods are more expensive than fast, processed foods. This book considers how this nutritional inequality is being addressed. It also looks at examples of healthy and unhealthy food, the health risks of a poor diet and strategies to help people eat better.

OUR SOURCES

Titles in the **issues** series are designed to function as educational resource books, providing a balanced overview of a specific subject.

The information in our books is comprised of facts, articles and opinions from many different sources, including:

♦ Newspaper reports and opinion pieces

♦ Website factsheets

♦ Magazine and journal articles

♦ Statistics and surveys

♦ Government reports

♦ Literature from special interest groups.

A NOTE ON CRITICAL EVALUATION

Because the information reprinted here is from a number of different sources, readers should bear in mind the origin of the text and whether the source is likely to have a particular bias when presenting information (or when conducting their research). It is hoped that, as you read about the many aspects of the issues explored in this book, you will critically evaluate the information presented.

It is important that you decide whether you are being presented with facts or opinions. Does the writer give a biased or unbiased report? If an opinion is being expressed, do you agree with the writer? Is there potential bias to the 'facts' or statistics behind an article?

ASSIGNMENTS

In the back of this book, you will find a selection of assignments designed to help you engage with the articles you have been reading and to explore your own opinions. Some tasks will take longer than others and there is a mixture of design, writing and research-based activities that you can complete alone or in a group.

FURTHER RESEARCH

At the end of each article we have listed its source and a website that you can visit if you would like to conduct your own research. Please remember to critically evaluate any sources that you consult and consider whether the information you are viewing is accurate and unbiased.

Useful Websites

www.achieveoxfordshire.org.uk

www.cam.ac.uk

www.eufic.org

www.foodfoundation.org.uk

www.foodnavigator.com

www.hriuk.org

www.metro.co.uk

www.nutrition.org.uk

www.shareaction.org

www.telegraph.co.uk

ww.thebackseateconomist.com

www.theconversation.com

www.thegrocer.co.uk

www.ukhsa.blog.gov.uk

www.who.int

www.york.ac.uk

Healthy Eating

Editor: Danielle Lobban

Volume 408

independence
educational publishers

First published by Independence Educational Publishers

The Studio, High Green

Great Shelford

Cambridge CB22 5EG

England

Copyright

Photocopy licence

ISBN-13: 978 1 86168 867 5

Printed in Great Britain

Zenith Print Group

Healthy diet

Key facts

♦ A healthy diet helps to protect against malnutrition in all its forms, as well as noncommunicable diseases (NCDs), including such as diabetes, heart disease, stroke and cancer.

♦ Unhealthy diet and lack of physical activity are leading global risks to health. Healthy dietary practices start early in life – breast-feeding fosters healthy growth and improves cognitive development, and may have longer term health benefits such as reducing the risk of becoming overweight or obese and developing NCDs later in life.

♦ Energy intake (calories) should be in balance with energy expenditure. To avoid unhealthy weight gain, total fat should not exceed 30% of total energy intake.[1, 2, 3] Intake of saturated fats should be less than 10% of total energy intake, and intake of trans-fats less than 1% of total energy intake, with a shift in fat consumption away from saturated fats and trans-fats to unsaturated fats,[3] and towards the goal of eliminating industrially-produced trans-fats.[4, 5, 6]

♦ Limiting intake of free sugars to less than 10% of total energy intake[2, 7] is part of a healthy diet. A further reduction to less than 5% of total energy intake is suggested for additional health benefits.[7]

♦ Keeping salt intake to less than 5g per day (equivalent to sodium intake of less than 2g per day) helps to prevent hypertension, and reduces the risk of heart disease and stroke in the adult population.[8]

♦ WHO Member States have agreed to reduce the global population's intake of salt by 30% by 2025; they have also agreed to halt the rise in diabetes and obesity in adults and adolescents as well as in childhood overweight by 2025.[9, 10]

Overview

Consuming a healthy diet throughout the life-course helps to prevent malnutrition in all its forms as well as a range of noncommunicable diseases (NCDs) and conditions. However, increased production of processed foods, rapid urbanization and changing lifestyles have led to a shift in dietary patterns. People are now consuming more foods high in energy, fats, free sugars and salt/sodium, and many people do not eat enough fruit, vegetables and other dietary fibre such as whole grains.

The exact make-up of a diversified, balanced and healthy diet will vary depending on individual characteristics (e.g. age, gender, lifestyle and degree of physical activity), cultural context, locally available foods and dietary customs. However, the basic principles of what constitutes a healthy diet remain the same.

For adults

A healthy diet includes the following:

♦ Fruit, vegetables, legumes (e.g. lentils and beans), nuts and whole grains (e.g. unprocessed maize, millet, oats, wheat and brown rice).

♦ At least 400g (i.e. five portions) of fruit and vegetables per day,[2] excluding potatoes, sweet potatoes, cassava and other starchy roots.

♦ Less than 10% of total energy intake from free sugars,[2, 7] which is equivalent to 50g (or about 12 level teaspoons) for a person of healthy body weight consuming about 2000 calories per day, but ideally is less than 5% of total energy intake for additional health benefits.[7] Free sugars are all sugars added to foods or drinks by the manufacturer, cook or consumer, as well as sugars naturally present in honey, syrups, fruit juices and fruit juice concentrates.

♦ Less than 30% of total energy intake from fats.[1,2,3] Unsaturated fats (found in fish, avocado and nuts, and in sunflower, soybean, canola and olive oils) are preferable to saturated fats (found in fatty meat, butter, palm and coconut oil, cream, cheese, ghee and lard) and trans-fats of all kinds, including both industrially-produced trans-fats (found in baked and fried foods, and pre-packaged snacks and foods, such as frozen pizza, pies, cookies, biscuits, wafers, and cooking oils and spreads) and ruminant trans-fats (found in meat and dairy foods from ruminant animals, such as cows, sheep, goats and camels). It is suggested that the intake of saturated fats be reduced to less than 10% of total energy intake and trans-fats to less than 1% of total energy intake.[5] In particular, industrially-produced trans-fats are not part of a healthy diet and should be avoided.[4, 6]

♦ Less than 5g of salt (equivalent to about one teaspoon) per day.[8] Salt should be iodized.

For infants and young children

In the first 2 years of a child's life, optimal nutrition fosters healthy growth and improves cognitive development. It also reduces the risk of becoming overweight or obese and developing NCDs later in life.

Advice on a healthy diet for infants and children is similar to that for adults, but the following elements are also important:

♦ Infants should be breast-fed exclusively during the first 6 months of life.

♦ Infants should be breast-fed continuously until 2 years of age and beyond.

♦ From 6 months of age, breast milk should be complemented with a variety of adequate, safe and nutrient-dense foods. Salt and sugars should not be added to complementary foods.

Practical advice on maintaining a healthy diet

Fruit and vegetables

Eating at least 400g, or five portions, of fruit and vegetables per day reduces the risk of NCDs[2] and helps to ensure an adequate daily intake of dietary fibre.

Fruit and vegetable intake can be improved by:

♦ always including vegetables in meals;

♦ eating fresh fruit and raw vegetables as snacks;

♦ eating fresh fruit and vegetables that are in season; and eating a variety of fruit and vegetables.

Fats

Reducing the amount of total fat intake to less than 30% of total energy intake helps to prevent unhealthy weight gain in the adult population.[1,2,3] Also, the risk of developing NCDs is lowered by:

♦ reducing saturated fats to less than 10% of total energy intake;

♦ reducing trans-fats to less than 1% of total energy intake; and

♦ replacing both saturated fats and trans-fats with unsaturated fats [2,3] – in particular, with polyunsaturated fats.

Fat intake, especially saturated fat and industrially-produced trans-fat intake, can be reduced by:

♦ steaming or boiling instead of frying when cooking;

♦ replacing butter, lard and ghee with oils rich in polyunsaturated fats, such as soybean, canola (rapeseed), corn, safflower and sunflower oils;

♦ eating reduced-fat dairy foods and lean meats, or trimming visible fat from meat; and

♦ limiting the consumption of baked and fried foods, and pre-packaged snacks and foods (e.g. doughnuts, cakes, pies, cookies, biscuits and wafers) that contain industrially-produced trans-fats.

Salt, sodium and potassium

Most people consume too much sodium through salt (corresponding to consuming an average of 9–12g of salt per day) and not enough potassium (less than 3.5g). High sodium intake and insufficient potassium intake contribute to high blood pressure, which in turn increases the risk of heart disease and stroke. [8,11]

Reducing salt intake to the recommended level of less than 5 g per day could prevent 1.7 million deaths each year. [12]

People are often unaware of the amount of salt they consume. In many countries, most salt comes from processed foods (e.g. ready meals; processed meats such as bacon, ham and salami; cheese; and salty snacks) or from foods consumed frequently in large amounts (e.g. bread). Salt is also added to foods during cooking (e.g. bouillon, stock cubes, soy sauce and fish sauce) or at the point of consumption (e.g. table salt).

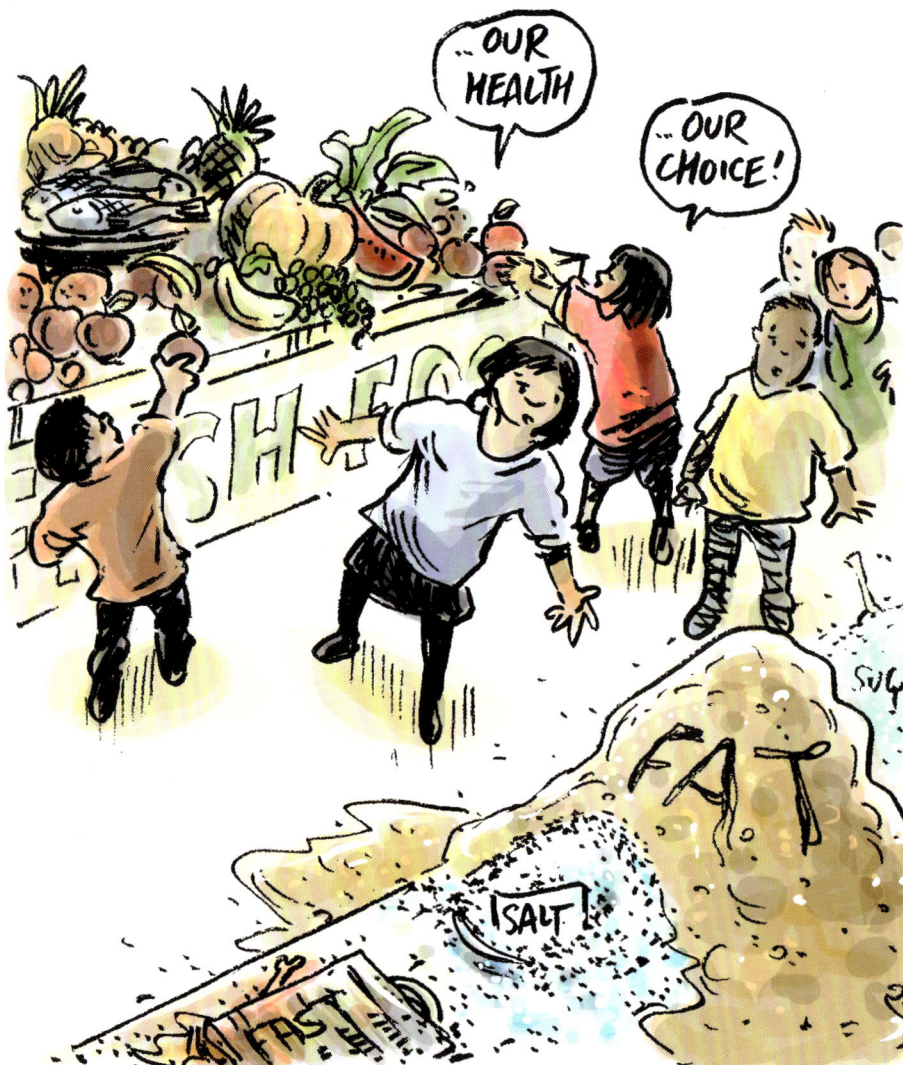

Salt intake can be reduced by:

- limiting the amount of salt and high-sodium condiments (e.g. soy sauce, fish sauce and bouillon) when cooking and preparing foods;

- not having salt or high-sodium sauces on the table;

- limiting the consumption of salty snacks; and

- choosing products with lower sodium content.

Some food manufacturers are reformulating recipes to reduce the sodium content of their products, and people should be encouraged to check nutrition labels to see how much sodium is in a product before purchasing or consuming it.

Potassium can mitigate the negative effects of elevated sodium consumption on blood pressure. Intake of potassium can be increased by consuming fresh fruit and vegetables.

Sugars

In both adults and children, the intake of free sugars should be reduced to less than 10% of total energy intake.[2,7] A reduction to less than 5% of total energy intake would provide additional health benefits. [7]

Consuming free sugars increases the risk of dental caries (tooth decay). Excess calories from foods and drinks high in free sugars also contribute to unhealthy weight gain, which can lead to overweight and obesity. Recent evidence also shows that free sugars influence blood pressure and serum lipids, and suggests that a reduction in free sugars intake reduces risk factors for cardiovascular diseases.[13]

Sugars intake can be reduced by:

- limiting the consumption of foods and drinks containing high amounts of sugars, such as sugary snacks, candies and sugar-sweetened beverages (i.e. all types of beverages containing free sugars – these include carbonated or non-carbonated soft drinks, fruit or vegetable juices and drinks, liquid and powder concentrates, flavoured water, energy and sports drinks, ready-to-drink tea, ready-to-drink coffee and flavoured milk drinks); and

- eating fresh fruit and raw vegetables as snacks instead of sugary snacks.

How to promote healthy diets

Diet evolves over time, being influenced by many social and economic factors that interact in a complex manner to shape individual dietary patterns. These factors include income, food prices (which will affect the availability and affordability of healthy foods), individual preferences and beliefs, cultural traditions, and geographical and environmental aspects (including climate change). Therefore, promoting a healthy food environment – including food systems that promote a diversified, balanced and healthy diet – requires the involvement of multiple sectors and stakeholders, including government, and the public and private sectors.

Governments have a central role in creating a healthy food environment that enables people to adopt and maintain healthy dietary practices. Effective actions by policy-makers to create a healthy food environment include the following:

- Creating coherence in national policies and investment plans – including trade, food and agricultural policies – to promote a healthy diet and protect public health through:
  - increasing incentives for producers and retailers to grow, use and sell fresh fruit and vegetables;
  - reducing incentives for the food industry to continue or increase production of processed foods containing high levels of saturated fats, trans-fats, free sugars and salt/sodium;
  - encouraging reformulation of food products to reduce the contents of saturated fats, trans-fats, free sugars and salt/sodium, with the goal of eliminating industrially-produced trans-fats;
  - implementing the WHO recommendations on the marketing of foods and non-alcoholic beverages to children;
  - establishing standards to foster healthy dietary practices through ensuring the availability of healthy, nutritious, safe and affordable foods in pre-schools, schools, other public institutions and the workplace;
  - exploring regulatory and voluntary instruments (e.g. marketing regulations and nutrition labelling policies), and economic incentives or disincentives (e.g. taxation and subsidies) to promote a healthy diet; and
  - encouraging transnational, national and local food services and catering outlets to improve the nutritional quality of their foods – ensuring the availability and affordability of healthy choices – and review portion sizes and pricing.

- Encouraging consumer demand for healthy foods and meals through:
  - promoting consumer awareness of a healthy diet;
  - developing school policies and programmes that encourage children to adopt and maintain a healthy diet;
  - educating children, adolescents and adults about nutrition and healthy dietary practices;
  - encouraging culinary skills, including in children through schools;
  - supporting point-of-sale information, including through nutrition labelling that ensures accurate, standardized and comprehensible information on nutrient contents in foods (in line with the Codex Alimentarius Commission guidelines), with the addition of front-of-pack labelling to facilitate consumer understanding; and
  - providing nutrition and dietary counselling at primary health-care facilities.

- Promoting appropriate infant and young child feeding practices through:
  - implementing the International Code of Marketing of Breast-milk Substitutes and subsequent relevant World Health Assembly resolutions;

- implementing policies and practices to promote protection of working mothers; and

- promoting, protecting and supporting breast-feeding in health services and the community, including through the Baby-friendly Hospital Initiative.

WHO response

The 'WHO Global Strategy on Diet, Physical Activity and Health'[14] was adopted in 2004 by the Health Assembly. The strategy called on governments, WHO, international partners, the private sector and civil society to take action at global, regional and local levels to support healthy diets and physical activity.

In 2010, the Health Assembly endorsed a set of recommendations on the marketing of foods and non-alcoholic beverages to children.[15] These recommendations guide countries in designing new policies and improving existing ones to reduce the impact on children of the marketing of foods and non-alcoholic beverages to children. WHO has also developed region-specific tools (such as regional nutrient profile models) that countries can use to implement the marketing recommendations.

In 2012, the Health Assembly adopted a 'Comprehensive Implementation Plan on Maternal, Infant and Young Child Nutrition' and six global nutrition targets to be achieved by 2025, including the reduction of stunting, wasting and overweight in children, the improvement of breast-feeding, and the reduction of anaemia and low birthweight.[9]

In 2013, the Health Assembly agreed to nine global voluntary targets for the prevention and control of NCDs. These targets include a halt to the rise in diabetes and obesity, and a 30% relative reduction in the intake of salt by 2025. The 'Global Action Plan for the Prevention and Control of Noncommunicable Diseases 2013–2020'[10] provides guidance and policy options for Member States, WHO and other United Nations agencies to achieve the targets.

With many countries now seeing a rapid rise in obesity among infants and children, in May 2014 WHO set up the Commission on Ending Childhood Obesity. In 2016, the Commission proposed a set of recommendations to successfully tackle childhood and adolescent obesity in different contexts around the world.[16]

In November 2014, WHO organized, jointly with the Food and Agriculture Organization of the United Nations (FAO), the Second International Conference on Nutrition (ICN2). ICN2 adopted the Rome Declaration on Nutrition,[17] and the Framework for Action[18] which recommends a set of policy options and strategies to promote diversified, safe and healthy diets at all stages of life. WHO is helping countries to implement the commitments made at ICN2.

In May 2018, the Health Assembly approved the 13th General Programme of Work (GPW13), which will guide the work of WHO in 2019–2023.[19] Reduction of salt/sodium intake and elimination of industrially-produced trans-fats from the food supply are identified in GPW13 as part of WHO's priority actions to achieve the aims of ensuring healthy lives and promote well-being for all at all ages. To support Member States in taking necessary actions to eliminate industrially-produced trans-fats, WHO has developed a road map for countries (the REPLACE action package) to help accelerate actions.[6]

References

(1) Hooper L, Abdelhamid A, Bunn D, Brown T, Summerbell CD, Skeaff CM. Effects of total fat intake on body weight. Cochrane Database Syst Rev. 2015; (8):CD011834.

(2) Diet, nutrition and the prevention of chronic diseases: report of a Joint WHO/FAO Expert Consultation. WHO Technical Report Series, No. 916. Geneva: World Health Organization; 2003.

(3) Fats and fatty acids in human nutrition: report of an expert consultation. FAO Food and Nutrition Paper 91. Rome: Food and Agriculture Organization of the United Nations; 2010.

(4) Nishida C, Uauy R. WHO scientific update on health consequences of trans fatty acids: introduction. Eur J Clin Nutr. 2009; 63 Suppl 2:S1–4.

(5) Guidelines: Saturated fatty acid and trans-fatty acid intake for adults and children. Geneva: World Health Organization; 2018 (Draft issued for public consultation in May 2018).

(6) REPLACE: An action package to eliminate industrially-produced trans-fatty acids. WHO/NMH/NHD/18.4. Geneva: World Health Organization; 2018.

(7) Guideline: Sugars intake for adults and children. Geneva: World Health Organization; 2015.

(8) Guideline: Sodium intake for adults and children. Geneva: World Health Organization; 2012.

(9) Comprehensive implementation plan on maternal, infant and young child nutrition. Geneva: World Health Organization; 2014.

(10) Global action plan for the prevention and control of NCDs 2013–2020. Geneva: World Health Organization; 2013.

(11) Guideline: Potassium intake for adults and children. Geneva: World Health Organization; 2012.

(12) Mozaffarian D, Fahimi S, Singh GM, Micha R, Khatibzadeh S, Engell RE et al. Global sodium consumption and death from cardiovascular causes. N Engl J Med. 2014; 371(7):624–34.

(13) Te Morenga LA, Howatson A, Jones RM, Mann J. Dietary sugars and cardiometabolic risk: systematic review and meta-analyses of randomized controlled trials of the effects on blood pressure and lipids. AJCN. 2014; 100(1): 65–79.

(14) Global strategy on diet, physical activity and health. Geneva: World Health Organization; 2004.

(15) Set of recommendations on the marketing of foods and non-alcoholic beverages to children. Geneva: World Health Organization; 2010.

(16) Report of the Commission on Ending Childhood Obesity. Geneva: World Health Organization; 2016.

(17) Rome Declaration on Nutrition. Second International Conference on Nutrition. Rome: Food and Agriculture Organization of the United Nations/ World Health Organization; 2014.

(18) Framework for Action. Second International Conference on Nutrition. Rome: Food and Agriculture Organization of the United Nations/World Health Organization; 2014.

(19) Thirteenth general programme of work, 2019–2023. Geneva: World Health Organization; 2018.

29 April 2020

How much water should you drink per day?

We can go for 50 days without food, but only two to three without water. Water is essential to the human body and we need about 2.5 litres of water a day.[1] Most of this will come from fluids but some from solid or liquid food.

The total of 2.5 litres per day is a rough estimate and depends on several factors:

- Age
- Sex
- Weight
- Height
- Level of physical activity
- Temperature & climate

Water in our body

The water content in our body diminishes as we age. Newborns have the most with 75% and the elderly the least with 55%. Adults have on average 60% of water in their body.[1,2]

So where exactly in the body is the water stored? One third is in our blood and between our cells, while the majority, two thirds, is in our cells.

If your body gets dehydrated, many bodily functions can be affected, because water regulates:[2]

- Body temperature
- Hormone regulation
- Energy expenditure stimulation
- Thickness of blood
- Skin moisture
- Cell longevity
- Positive digestion
- Cushion function for the spinal cord, brain and eyes
- Waste product elimination

Our body loses water constantly through breath, sweat, urine and faeces.[1] We lose even more water if we are ill, through vomiting and diarrhoea, so this increases our risk of dehydration.

How thirsty are you?

Because water is so important for our survival our body has a very good way of letting us know if we are becoming dehydrated. Thirst. If you feel thirsty, you know you need to drink.

Have you ever wondered how your body knows when you're dehydrated? In our brain, receptors measure blood consistency and react if it gets thinner. As a result, a hormone called vasopressin gets released into our system. Vasopressin makes sure we keep more water in our body, by retaining water in our kidneys and igniting the feeling of thirst.[1]

If you want to double check your hydration status, a simple way is to look at the colour of your urine. Light yellow means you're hydrated, but if it turns dark yellow you are dehydrated.

Dehydration, which happens when the body does not have enough water, is very dangerous. If we lose just 1% of our body water, we have decreased power for exercise, decreased temperature control in our body and less appetite. At 5% water loss, our mental performance decreases; with trouble concentrating, irritability, sleepiness, and often headaches. If we lose more than 8% of our water, we could actually die.[1]

Have you ever been so concentrated or busy you simply forgot to drink? Symptoms that might show up are:[1]

- Dry, sticky mouth
- Muscle cramps
- Headache
- Dry skin
- Tiredness
- Loss of concentration

Your urine colour says a lot about your hydration status

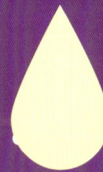

hydrated
keep drinking at the same rate

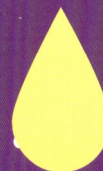

mildly hydrated
drink a glass of water now

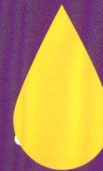

dehydrated
drink 2-3 glasses of water now

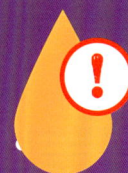

very dehydrated
drink a large botttle of water immediately

Stay hydrated

The European Food Safety Authority (EFSA) proposes the following guidelines for healthy total water intake.[1]

Group	Recommended total water intake (per day)
Infants (0-6 months old)	100 – 190 ml per kg bodyweight, from breastmilk
Infants (6-12 months old)	0.8 – 1.0 litres
Children (1-2 years old)	1.1 – 1.2 litres
Children (2-3 years old)	1.3 litres
Children (4-8 years)	1.6 litres
Boys (9-13 years old)	2.1 litres
Girls (9-13 years old)	1.9 litres
Adult men (older than 14 years)	2.5 litres
Adult women (older than 14 years)	2.0 litres

Drinking this much water seems like a lot but remember that these are recommendations for our overall water intake, which includes the water we take in through our food.

As a rule of thumb, 20-30% of the water we need comes from our food. Eating a balanced diet with a wide variety of fruit and vegetables can already help us stay hydrated.

The recommended intake of water we need to drink would look more like this:

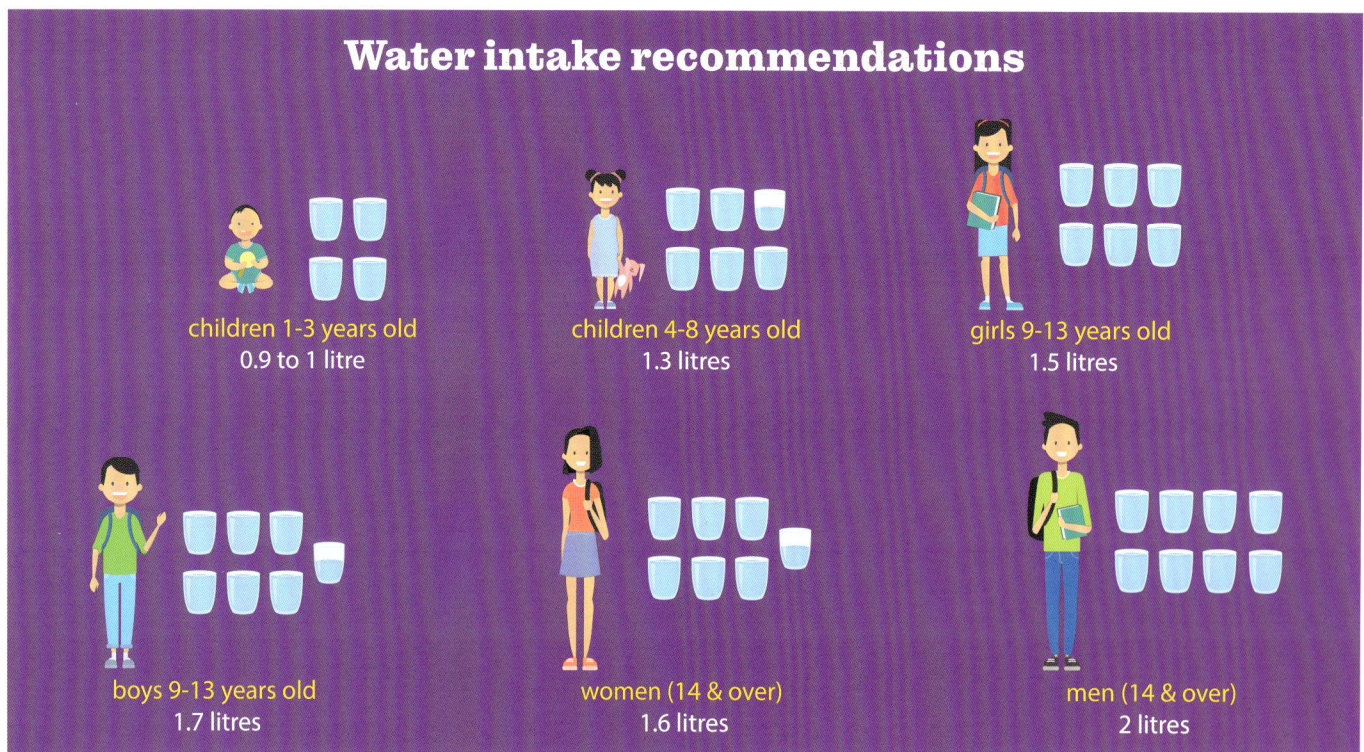

Water intake recommendations

children 1-3 years old
0.9 to 1 litre

children 4-8 years old
1.3 litres

girls 9-13 years old
1.5 litres

boys 9-13 years old
1.7 litres

women (14 & over)
1.6 litres

men (14 & over)
2 litres

Spark up your water!

Why not try...

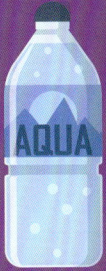

sparkling water

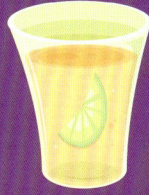

unsweetened flavoured water

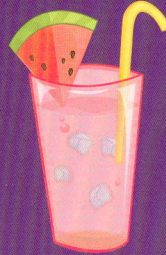

fruit or citrus infused water

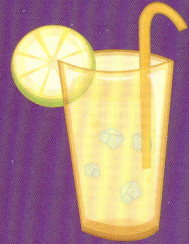

unsweetened iced tea

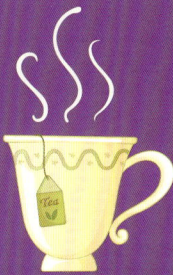

unsweetened brewed tea

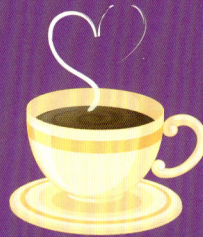

brewed coffee

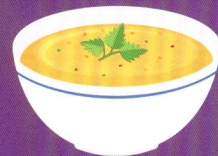

homemade soup

Too much water

The 'more is not always better' rule does apply when it comes to water. You can get water intoxication, hyponatremia, from drinking too much. This is a condition of over hydration causing salt levels to lower in the blood and excessive water to move inside cells which may lead to lung congestion and loss of muscle cells.[1] Therefore, it's recommended to always add a bit of salt to your water when you have to drink an exceptional amount. For example, we need to drink a lot, especially when exercising in a hot climate and for long periods of time (e.g. long-distance cycling and marathons) as a lot of fluid is lost through sweat. Sweat loss also means salt loss, which can cause cramps and exhaustion. Therefore, it's important to drink isotonic drinks, which contain sodium and correspond with the composition of our body fluids.[1]

Best sources of water

It's easy to drink more fluids on a daily basis. Not only plain water but all sorts of drinks can keep you hydrated.

TIP: If you don't like the taste of plain water there are some ways you can make it more enjoyable. A refreshing way is to add either ice cubes, slices of lemon, cucumber, some mint or berries.

When we open the tap, we have drinking water at our disposal at any time. Water is essential to our lives, but we might take its presence for granted. Governmental authorities regulate the safety of water used for human consumption (e.g. as drinking water or in food production).

The quality of the water depends on its source. For safety, tap water needs to be filtered multiple times, to bind dirt, and only a minimal amount of disinfectant (e.g. chlorine) can be added to kill any remaining microorganisms.

Make hydration easy

Some easy practical solutions can prevent dehydration. Always carry a refillable water bottle with you and challenge yourself to finish it by the end of the day. This makes sure you always have easy access to water and don't need to buy plastic bottles. Also, make sure to have water near you when you are at work. To make drinking even easier (and more fun) you can use a reusable straw. Finally, there are certain apps that can help you keep track of your water intake and send you reminders to drink throughout the day.

References

1. European food Safety Authority (EFSA) (2010). Scientific Opinion on Dietary Reference Values for water. EFSA Journal, 18-38.
2. EU Science Hub (2019). Water. European Commission.

26 March 2020

www.eufic.org

New data reveals how our diets are changing over time

By Alison Tedstone

We now know more than we ever have about what makes a good, balanced diet and the ways in which different nutrients impact our health.

Analysis of the burden of disease in England highlights the importance of a healthy diet and weight on risk of preventable diseases such as heart disease and some cancers.

The National Diet and Nutrition Survey has been running since 2008 and provides a crucial insight into how our dietary habits are changing over time.

The survey works by asking 1,000 people each year (500 adults and 500 children) about their dietary habits over a four-day period, with the sample designed to be representative of the UK population.

Blood and urine samples are taken to help us understand the level of different nutrients that people are consuming through what they eat and drink. The study is carried out by a consortium comprising NatCen Social Research and the National Institute of Health Research Cambridge Biomedical Research Centre.

It is the only survey in the UK to provide detailed information on food and nutrition intake within the population, with findings made available to researchers around the world.

Results are published every two to three years. Earlier this month we published the latest data from 2016/2017 to 2018/2019, giving us a snapshot of the state of the nation's diet during this time.

Overall, there are positive signs that our diets may be becoming healthier, though there remain some concerning trends.

Eating too much sugar is a major cause of tooth decay and excess weight. While sugar consumption remains too high, since 2008 there has been a steady decline in sugar intake in both children and adults.

There isn't a single factor at play here, but it is certainly in part thanks to a reduction in sugar sweetened soft drink consumption as people's tastes have changed and as more manufacturers have offered low sugar alternatives.

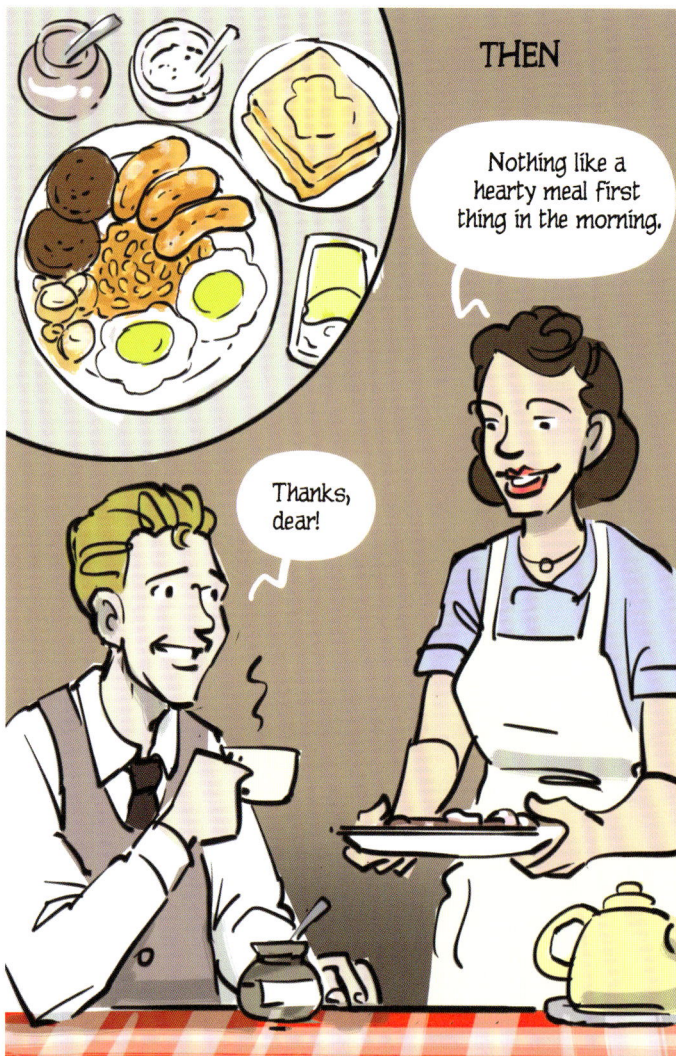

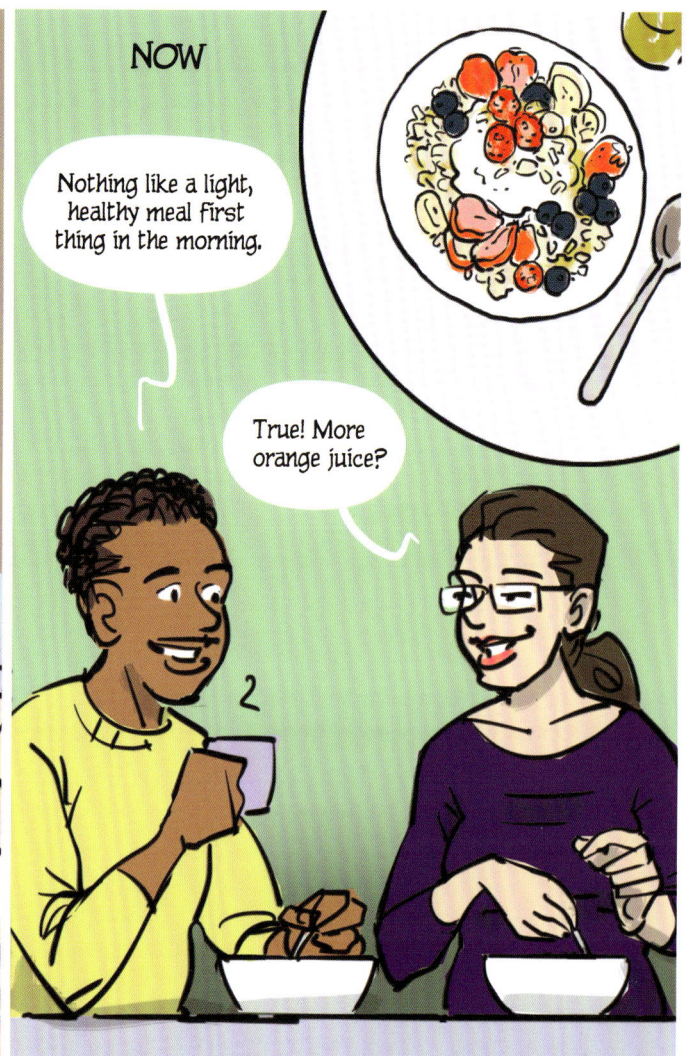

This is an encouraging sign that government-led initiatives to reduce sugar intake are having a positive impact on our diets, and dovetails with our analysis of changes in the sugar levels of drinks, carried out as part of the sugar reduction programme.

However, further data shows that while consumption of sugary drinks has fallen, there has been no decline in sweet confectionery and chocolate consumption, with intake even going up in some groups.

While sugar consumption remains too high in both children and adults, the decreasing trend overall is encouraging.

There has also been a fall in red and processed meat consumption over the past decade, most likely for environmental and health reasons. Significantly, all adults now consume, on average, below the maximum recommended daily intake of red and processed meat (70g per day).

This is good news because we know that while red meat can form part of a healthy diet evidence indicates that eating too much can increase your risk of developing bowel cancer.

While there are positive signs that our dietary habits are changing for the better there do remain several concerning trends.

It is particularly concerning that saturated fat intake looks to be increasing in some groups, as this a major contributor to high cholesterol and therefore heart disease. SACN's advice remains that saturated fats should be reduced to no more than about 10% of dietary energy.

While it is not possible to say definitively why this is happening, we do know there has been a big increase in popularity for lower-carb diets over recent years, many of which promote the consumption of higher-fat foods over those that are higher in wholegrain, starchy carbohydrate.

Average intakes of fibre, which is important for our digestive health, are still far below the recommended daily amount, with little sign of any meaningful change since 2008.

The latest data on salt intake for adults shows that average salt intake in 2020 was still higher (8.4g) than the recommended intake of 6g per day. While salt intake was been decreasing slowly over time, this decrease has slowed since 2014.

The latest NDNS also tells us that most people are still not eating the recommended 5 portions of fresh fruit and vegetables a day. Children aged 11 to 18 still only eat around 3 portions a day, though there has been a slight increase in consumption since 2014-16.

The data also gives us an understanding of lesser-known nutrient intakes that remain vital for our health.

One concerning trend is the steady decline in blood folate levels recorded by the survey since 2008, especially in women defined as being within childbearing age.

Having sufficient folic acid has been proven to significantly reduce the risks of the neural tube defect spina bifida occurring in pregnancy.

It is unclear why intake is declining but it is important that we try and reverse this trend. We know that food fortification can play an important role here: fortifying flour with folic acid is an effective and safe measure to reduce the number of pregnancies affected by neural tube defects. The Department of Health and Social Care have consulted on adding folic acid to flour and we support this.

The data also reminds us that most people do not get enough vitamin D, which is vital for bone and muscle health.

With many of us having been indoors more than usual this year, it's especially important for everyone to take a daily vitamin D supplement containing 10 micrograms (400IU) as we go into the winter months, particularly vulnerable groups such as the elderly, those who don't get outside and those with dark skin. Clinically vulnerable groups will be eligible for free vitamin D supplements throughout the winter period, starting in January.

While vitamin D plays an important role in our overall health, there is currently not enough evidence to support taking vitamin D solely to prevent or treat COVID-19.

Overall, the NDNS reminds us of the importance of promoting the benefits of a healthy, balanced diet as a foundation to good health.

While people's diets may be improving in some areas, two thirds of the population remain overweight or are living with obesity and poor diets remain one of the leading causes of disease such as cancer, heart disease and type 2 diabetes. As we said in the summer, there is now stark evidence that living with obesity also increases the risk of severe COVID-19. This may also explain some of the inequities seen in COVID-19 risk across society.

There is no silver bullet to this challenge but encouraging and promoting healthier choices is of course a key factor. PHE is clear in its support for commitments set out by the Government to reduce the advertising and promotion of less healthy foods, to better support healthier choices.

We also are committed to continuing to monitor the nation's diet and the progress of the food industry in their efforts on reducing sugar, salt and calories in everyday products.

Avoiding excess calories and eating more fruit and vegetables, fibre and oily fish and less sugar, salt and saturated fat will help everyone lower their risk of long term health problems.

21 December 2020

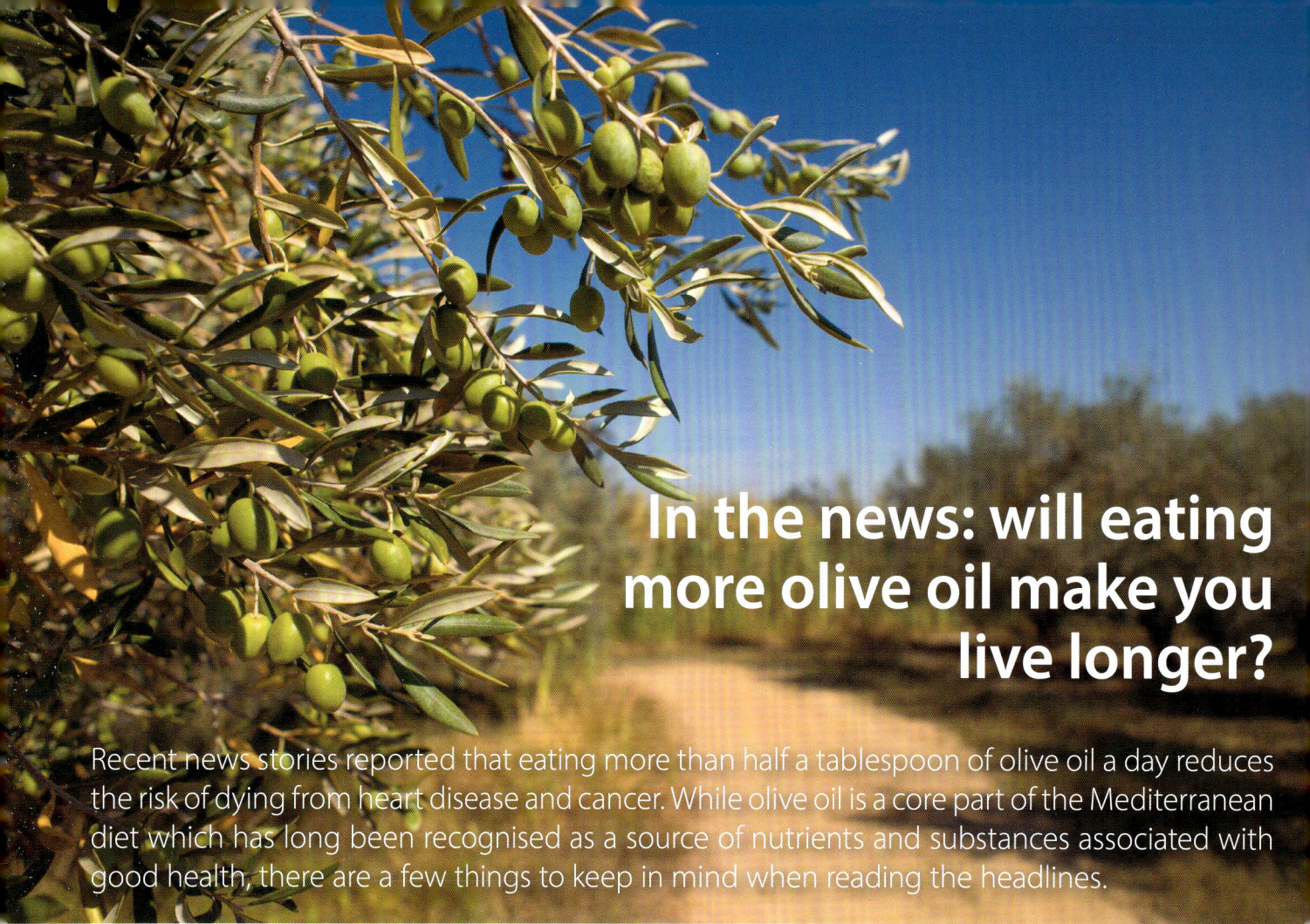

In the news: will eating more olive oil make you live longer?

Recent news stories reported that eating more than half a tablespoon of olive oil a day reduces the risk of dying from heart disease and cancer. While olive oil is a core part of the Mediterranean diet which has long been recognised as a source of nutrients and substances associated with good health, there are a few things to keep in mind when reading the headlines.

The study behind the headlines

The study behind the news used data from two older studies that started in the 70's and 80's and followed the diet, lifestyle and health of more than 90,000 participants (around 60,000 women and 30,000 men) over almost 30 years. Researchers then analysed the data specifically to look at the link between olive oil consumption and deaths.

The intake of fats and oils changed over time among participants, with average olive oil consumption increasing and margarine consumption decreasing.

Researchers found that increased olive oil consumption was linked to a lower risk of death overall and by specific causes. More specifically, they observed that participants that had higher intakes of olive oil (over 7 grams a day or half a tablespoon) had 19% less risk of dying from any cause. They were also 19% less likely to die from cardiovascular disease and 17% less likely to die from cancer.

Consistent risk reductions were also seen for deaths from degenerative brain diseases such as Alzheimer's disease and respiratory diseases.

The researchers concluded that replacing margarine, butter, mayonnaise and other dairy fat with olive oil could decrease death risk. However, there was no evidence that olive oil was preferable to other vegetable oils.

Which factors to consider when looking at the study conclusions?

It's difficult to fully ensure that olive oil consumption was the only dietary and lifestyle factor affecting the study's result.

For example, researchers found that people who consumed more olive oil also tended to have a healthier overall diet and were more physically active. Therefore, it's difficult to fully ensure that the influence of other lifestyle factors is completely removed from the analysis and so quantify with certainty the direct independent influence of a single factor such as olive oil.

Food frequency questionnaires may not give the full picture of how much and what type of olive oil is consumed.

Because food questionnaires depend on people's memory and subjective assessment of portion sizes, it may be difficult for people to accurately estimate their daily consumption of olive oil or other fats across different types of uses (for example, for baking or frying, added to salads or bread, etc.), which may fluctuate over time. The study also did not account for different types and quality of olive oil (for example, refined olive oil or extra virgin olive oil) which may have greater or lesser health benefits.

'Over half a tablespoon of olive oil a day' may not be necessary as benefits were also seen for smaller intakes.

Although the study found that a higher olive oil consumption was associated with a lower risk for all-cause, cardiovascular and cancer mortality, it's hard to be sure of the required intake level. Significant risk reductions were also seen with a daily intake of less than a teaspoon of olive oil.

The study only considered a specific US population and may not be representative of other populations, ethnicities and cultures.

This was a large study but included only middle-aged US health professionals in the 1970s-80s, mostly female and of 98% white ethnicity. More so, the changes in diets and lifestyle over the years add to the difficulty of understanding if the suggested olive oil intakes would have the same potential health influence today.

What do the authorities advise?

◆ WHO recommends that less than 30% of our energy intake comes from fats, and that unsaturated fats found in vegetable oils (such as olive, sunflower, canola and soybean oils) are preferable to saturated fats from animal products such as butter, cream, cheese, ghee and lard.[1]

◆ Specific recommendations for the consumption and use of different types of fat and oil varies between EU countries. Some countries quantify amounts or recommend overall categories or specific types of oil. Most say to limit saturated or animal fats and to opt for unsaturated or 'high quality' vegetable oils. Some countries such as Spain, Greece, Portugal, Romania, Malta, Cyprus and Croatia specify a preference for olive oil.[2]

References:

1. Guasch-Ferré M et al. (2022). Consumption of Olive Oil and Risk of Total and Cause-Specific Mortality Among U.S. Adults. Journal of American College of Cardiology 79(2), 101–112.

2. World Health Organisation (2015 updated). Healthy Diet Factsheet No 394.

3. EU Joint Research Centre. Health Promotion & Disease Prevention – Food-based Dietary Guidelines in Europe. Accessed on 16 Jan. 2022

19 January 2022

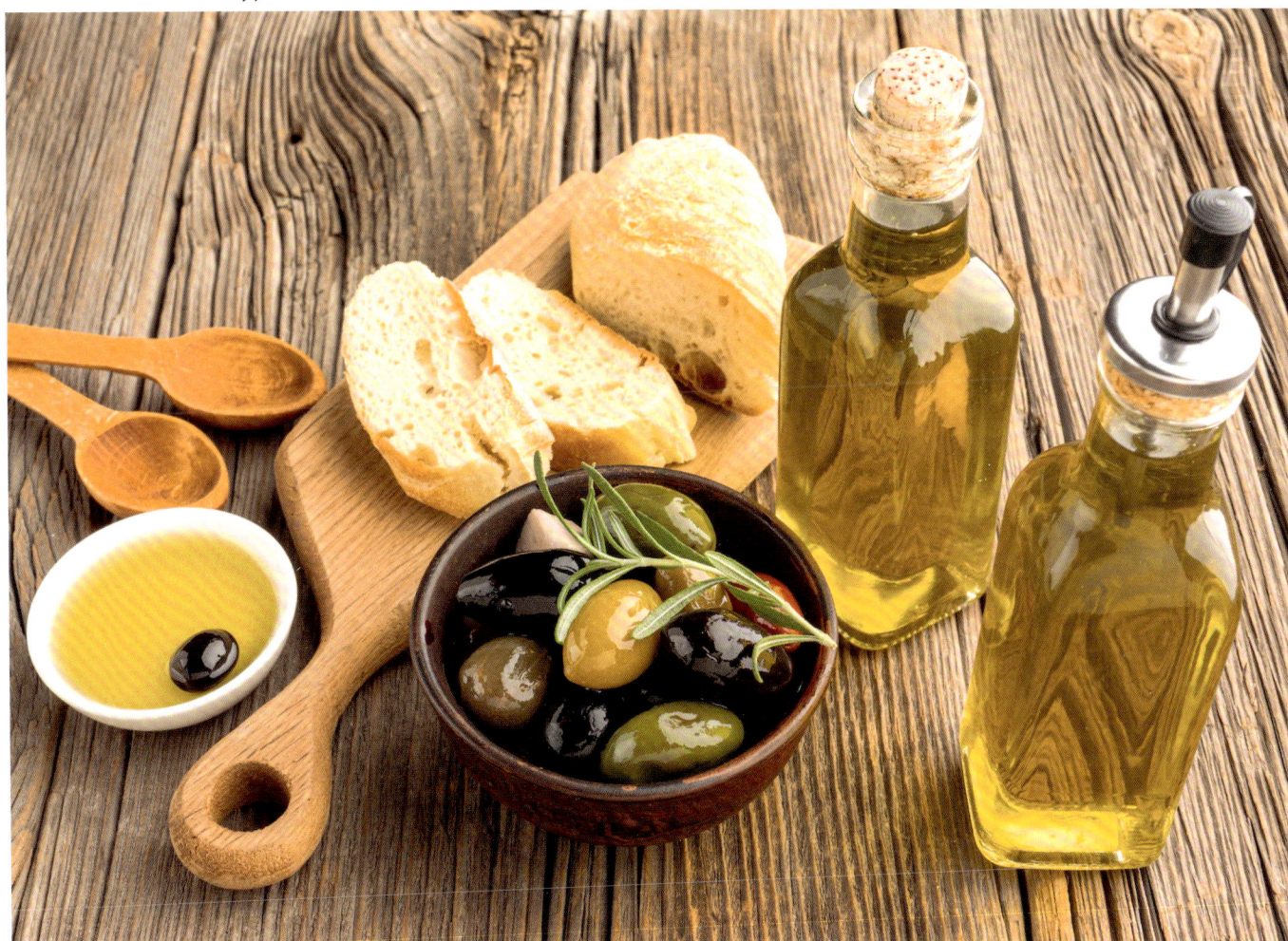

6 foods you thought were unhealthy

By The Healthy Eating Hub and Heart Research Institute

There is often conflicting information about whether a food is good for you and your heart, and if it should be added to your diet or avoided.

To start with, most foods require a context which can be used to help define whether or not its consumption is healthy. It's important to look at the bigger picture and assess a food within the whole diet – not just on its own, in isolation.

For example, carrots are commonly regarded as being healthy. They contain fibre, beta-carotene (converted into vitamin A by the body), vitamin C and other antioxidants and phytochemicals. Eating one to two carrots per day, as part of a balanced diet, is a healthy thing to do. However, if all you ate was carrots or you ate kilos of them every day, that would be unhealthy.

The main point here is that health (from a dietary perspective) is not the result of eating one type of food. It's the result of eating a variety of different, health-promoting foods consistently each day.

So in this context, here are six foods that have been sorely misunderstood.

Tofu

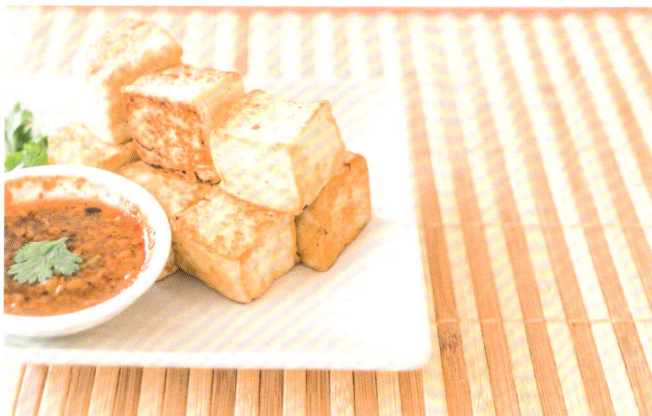

Soy products have often been blamed for poor health due to the presence of chemicals that are similar in structure to human reproductive hormones. Claims have also been made that the way soy is farmed and processed poses a risk to our health as well. Food regulation laws are very different across countries, which is the basis for some of this conflicting information. In addition, the 'evidence' for these claims is often taken out of context or from a poorly conducted study.

Tip: A serving of tofu three to four times per week, for example, is perfectly healthy and can be a great protein source, particularly for vegetarians or vegans. Tofu is versatile and with a bit of practice you can create lots of different, satisfying meals.

Nuts

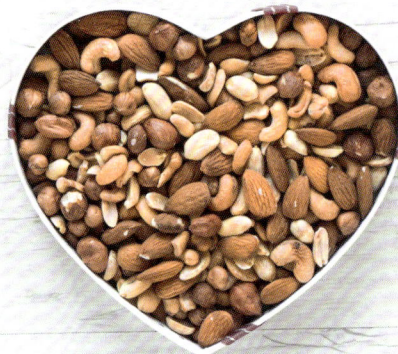

The fear of eating nuts most likely dates back to the low-fat era of the 80s and 90s. Nuts are rich in fats, among other nutrients, and as such are energy dense. This means that only a small serving can contain higher amounts of energy when compared to other foods.

Old school weight-loss programs saw this energy density as a problem and warned their clients against eating these foods, particularly for weight loss.

What these recommendations fail to recognise, again, is the context. Yes, if you consume too many nuts day-to-day, you may exceed your energy needs and find it difficult to lose weight. However, a small handful, consumed as part of a balanced diet, is perfectly fine.

Tip: Plenty of evidence suggests that due to the types of fat found in nuts, not to mention the dietary fibre, vitamins and minerals, that nuts are cardio-protective – meaning they decrease your risk of heart disease.

Wholegrain bread

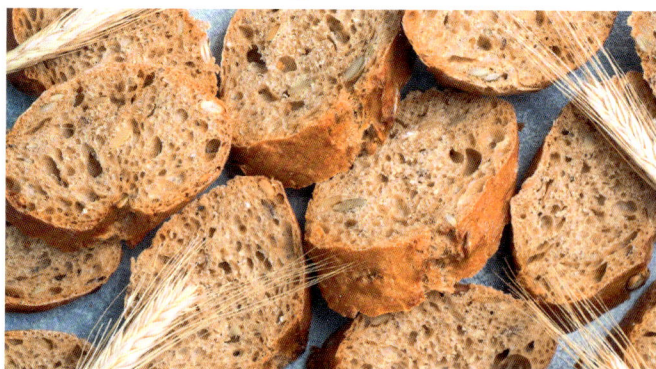

Often lumped into the white bread and refined carb basket, wholegrain bread, despite its fibre and nutrient content, is commonly thought of as unhealthy. You don't want to build your whole diet out of bread, but including a couple of slices

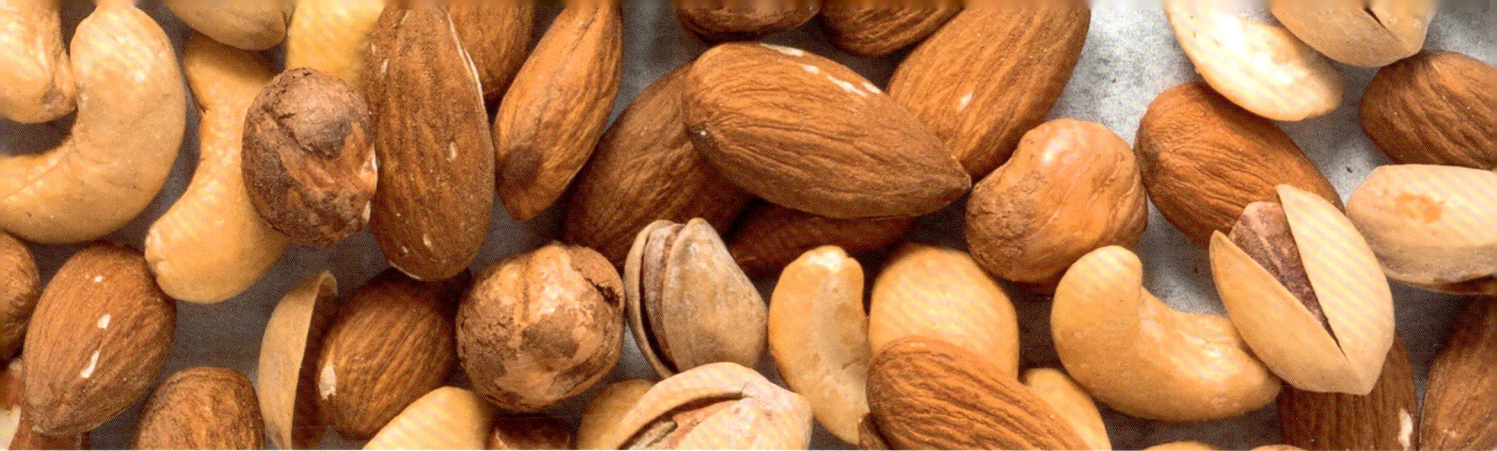

in your day can be a great way to get an important amount of dietary fibre, B vitamins and complex carbohydrates.

Tip: Serve wholegrain bread with protein and vegetables and you've got a winner of a balanced meal.

Eggs

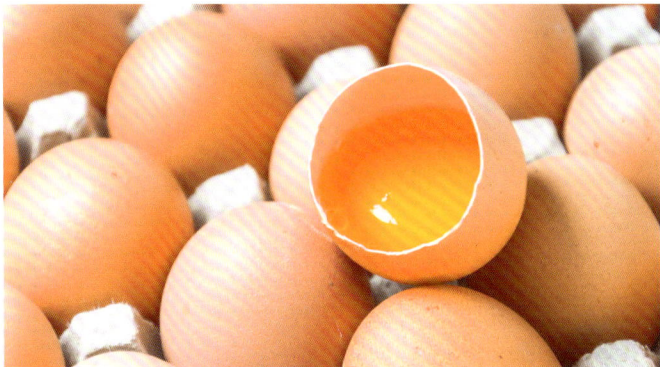

Eggs are a great source of protein and fat, along with other vitamins and minerals. Again, you don't want to build your whole diet out of eggs (which would make you rather gassy and backed up) but including one or two per day is perfectly healthy.

Tip: Eggs on wholegrain bread make a filling breakfast that will get you through the morning.

Bananas

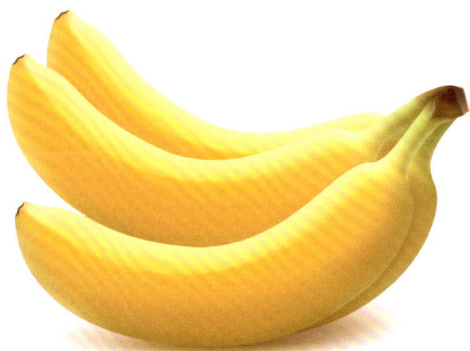

Bananas are a great source of dietary fibre for a healthy gut and carbohydrate (in the form of sugar) for energy, while only containing a smidgen more than other fruits. They are also full of potassium and other vitamins and minerals. Experts recommend that two serves of fruit per day is sufficient for most of us. If your day consists of minimal activity, sticking to a maximum of two serves of fruit per day (including bananas) is a good idea.

Tip: 1 serve of fruit = 1 banana or 1 apple or 1 cup of berries. So, don't build your whole diet out of bananas, but certainly include them daily as part of your healthy, balanced day.

Milk

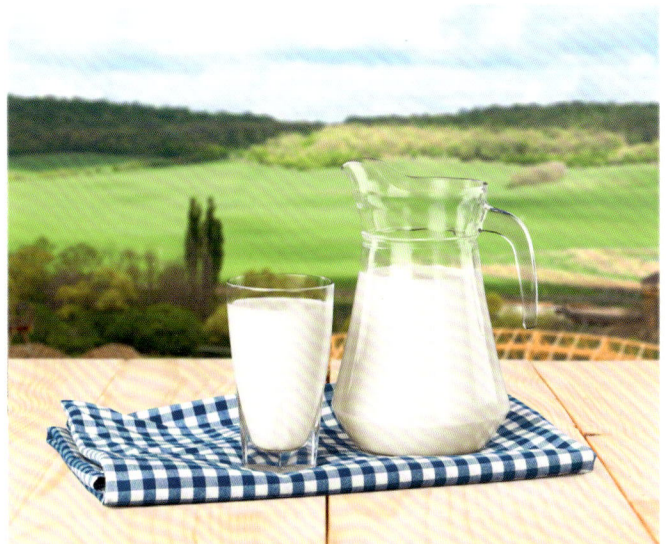

While you don't have to drink milk if you don't want to, don't stop drinking it because you've been told it's unhealthy or unnatural. It's not a good idea to build your whole diet out of dairy, but a milky coffee or bowl of cereal and milk per day is fine.

Tip: As part of a healthy diet, milk offers protein, calcium, vitamin B12, potassium and other nutrients.

2022

This article was written by an Accredited Practicing Dietitian from The Healthy Eating Hub. The Healthy Eating Hub is a team of university-qualified nutritionists and dietitians who are passionate about helping people develop long term healthy eating habits through offering evidence-based and practical nutrition advice that people can put into practice straight away.

www.hriuk.org

What you eat can reprogram your genes – an expert explains the emerging science of nutrigenomics

An article from *The Conversation*.

THE CONVERSATION

By Monica Dus, Assistant Professor of Molecular, Cellular, and Developmental Biology, University of Michigan

People typically think of food as calories, energy and sustenance. However, the latest evidence suggests that food also 'talks' to our genome, which is the genetic blueprint that directs the way the body functions down to the cellular level.

This communication between food and genes may affect your health, physiology and longevity. The idea that food delivers important messages to an animal's genome is the focus of a field known as nutrigenomics. This is a discipline still in its infancy, and many questions remain cloaked in mystery. Yet already, we researchers have learned a great deal about how food components affect the genome.

I am a molecular biologist who researches the interactions among food, genes and brains in the effort to better understand how food messages affect our biology. The efforts of scientists to decipher this transmission of information could one day result in healthier and happier lives for all of us. But until then, nutrigenomics has unmasked at least one important fact: Our relationship with food is far more intimate than we ever imagined.

The interaction of food and genes

If the idea that food can drive biological processes by interacting with the genome sounds astonishing, one need look no further than a beehive to find a proven and perfect example of how this happens. Worker bees labor nonstop, are sterile and live only a few weeks. The queen bee, sitting deep inside the hive, has a life span that lasts for years and a fecundity so potent she gives birth to an entire colony.

And yet, worker and queen bees are genetically identical organisms. They become two different life forms because of the food they eat. The queen bee feasts on royal jelly; worker bees feed on nectar and pollen. Both foods provide energy, but royal jelly has an extra feature: its nutrients can unlock the genetic instructions to create the anatomy and physiology of a queen bee.

So how is food translated into biological instructions? Remember that food is composed of macronutrients. These include carbohydrates – or sugars – proteins and fat. Food also contains micronutrients such as vitamins and minerals. These compounds and their breakdown products can trigger genetic switches that reside in the genome.–

Like the switches that control the intensity of the light in your house, genetic switches determine how much of a certain gene product is produced. Royal jelly, for instance, contains compounds that activate genetic controllers to form the queen's organs and sustain her reproductive ability. In humans and mice, byproducts of the amino acid methionine, which are abundant in meat and fish, are known to influence genetic dials that are important for cell growth and division. And vitamin C plays a role in keeping us healthy by protecting the genome from oxidative damage; it also promotes the function of cellular pathways that can repair the genome if it does get damaged.

Depending on the type of nutritional information, the genetic controls activated and the cell that receives them, the messages in food can influence wellness, disease risk and even life span. But it's important to note that to date, most of these studies have been conducted in animal models, like bees.

Interestingly, the ability of nutrients to alter the flow of genetic information can span across generations. Studies show that in humans and animals, the diet of grandparents influences the activity of genetic switches and the disease risk and mortality of grandchildren.

Cause and effect

One interesting aspect of thinking of food as a type of biological information is that it gives new meaning to the idea of a food chain. Indeed, if our bodies are influenced by what we have eaten – down to a molecular level – then what the food we consume 'ate' also could affect our genome. For example, compared to milk from grass-fed cows, the milk from grain-fed cattle has different amounts and types of fatty acids and vitamins C and A . So when humans drink these different types of milk, their cells also receive different nutritional messages.

Similarly, a human mother's diet changes the levels of fatty acids as well as vitamins such as B-6, B-12 and folate that are found in her breast milk. This could alter the type of nutritional messages reaching the baby's own genetic switches, although whether or not this has an effect on the child's development is, at the moment, unknown.

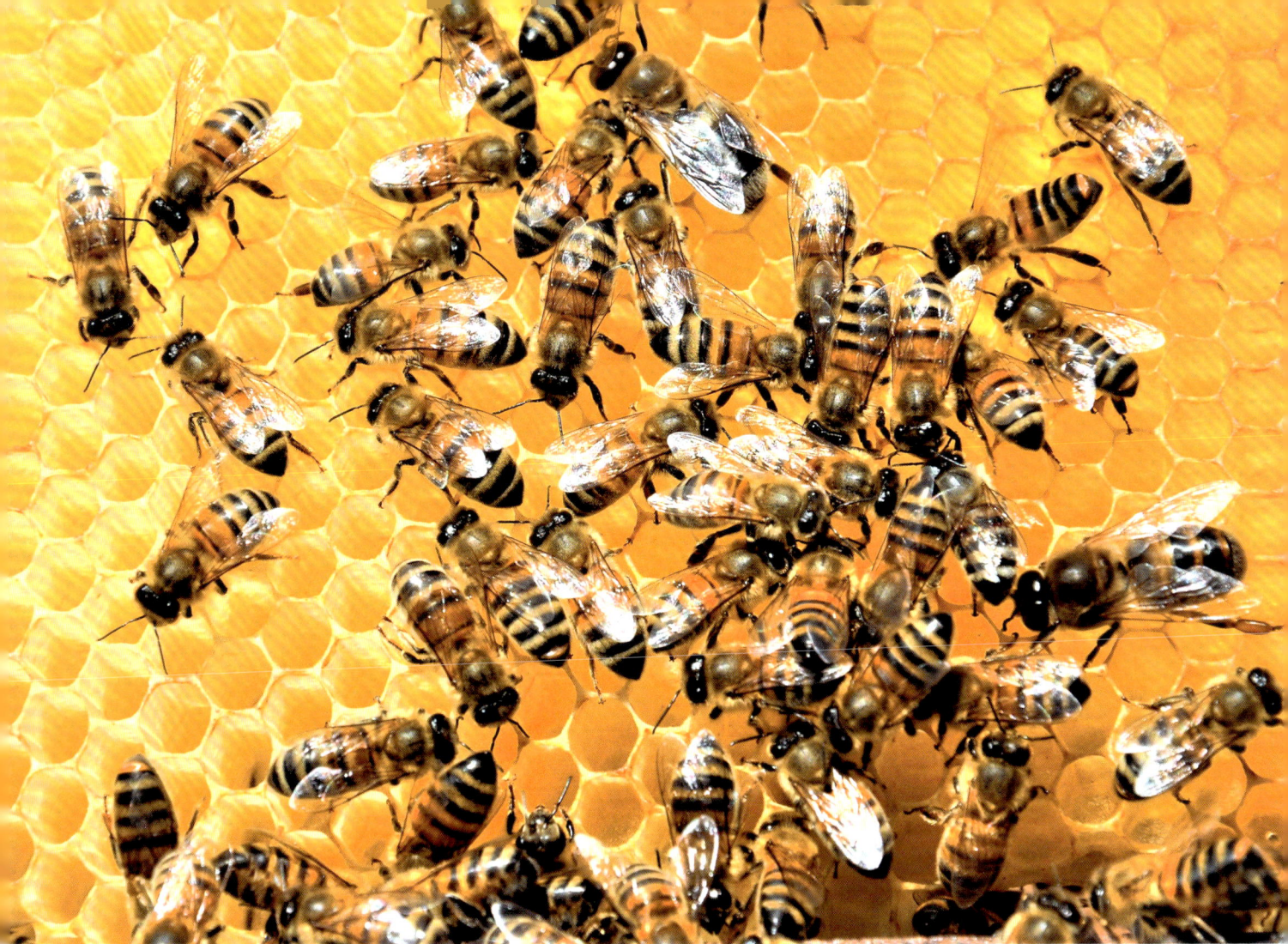

And, maybe unbeknownst to us, we too are part of this food chain. The food we eat doesn't tinker with just the genetic switches in our cells, but also with those of the microorganisms living in our guts, skin and mucosa. One striking example: In mice, the breakdown of short-chain fatty acids by gut bacteria alters the levels of serotonin, a brain chemical messenger that regulates mood, anxiety and depression, among other processes.

Food additives and packaging

Added ingredients in food can also alter the flow of genetic information inside cells. Breads and cereals are enriched with folate to prevent birth defects caused by deficiencies of this nutrient. But some scientists hypothesize that high levels of folate in the absence of other naturally occurring micronutrients such as vitamin B-12 could contribute to the higher incidence of colon cancer in Western countries, possibly by affecting the genetic pathways that control growth.

This could also be true with chemicals found in food packaging. Bisphenol A, or BPA, a compound found in plastic, turns on genetic dials in mammals that are critical to development, growth and fertility. For example, some researchers suspect that, in both humans and animal models, BPA influences the age of sexual differentiation and decreases fertility by making genetic switches more likely to turn on.

All of these examples point to the possibility that the genetic information in food could arise not just from its molecular composition – the amino acids, vitamins and the like – but also from the agricultural, environmental and economic policies of a country, or the lack of them.

Scientists have only recently begun decoding these genetic food messages and their role in health and disease. We researchers still don't know precisely how nutrients act on genetic switches, what their rules of communication are and how the diets of past generations influence their progeny. Many of these studies have so far been done only in animal models, and much remains to be worked out about what the interactions between food and genes mean for humans.

What is clear though, is that unraveling the mysteries of nutrigenomics is likely to empower both present and future societies and generations.

1 March 2022

The case for processed foods: 'Zero processing doesn't work for today's food choices'

With backlash mounting over ultra-processed foods, a research professor from Ghent University has balanced out the argument – making a strong case for processing where appropriate.

By Flora Southey

At a time when 'clean label' and 'natural' foods are the trendiest on-shelf, and growing scientific evidence points to links between ultra-processed foods and health risks, it is unsurprising that processed foods are falling out of favour.

According to a 2020 survey by the European Consumer Organisation (BEUC), foods that are 'minimal processed, traditional' matter to consumers. Such foods are most valued by consumers in Portugal, Greece and Lithuania, who associate them with 'sustainable food'.

In another survey, undertaken by L.E.K Consulting, consumers said the most important claim when purchasing food and drink was 'no artificial ingredients', followed by 'no preservatives'. In fourth place was a preference for the 'all natural' claim.

Yet according to research professor at Ghent University Andreja Rajkovic, processed foods are not wholly deserving of their bad reputation, and should not be perceived unilaterally as either 'friends or foes'.

Rather, at the European Food Information Council's (EUFIC) Processed Foods Symposium last week, the microbial food safety expert argued that certain processed foods more than merit their place in today's society.

What does food processing bring to the table?

At a personal level, Rajkovic himself opts for a minimally processed, clean label diet.

However, acknowledging that adhering to such a diet requires both time and money, his professional opinion supports food processing where appropriate. In fact, Rajkovic argues that food processing brings a great number of benefits to society.

Amongst the positive reasons for processing food, the research professor counted its ability to reduce food spoilage, extend shelf-life, and increase food safety.

In this respect, processing food also helps reduce food waste, he explained. 'A large proportion of food produced never actually gets eaten, but is thrown away – either through the processing [stage] or during household storage.'

Processing can also be used as a tool to modify the flavour, texture, aroma, colour or form of food. It can transform an ingredient, or a matrix of ingredients, into something that is 'palatable, eatable, and appealing to the consumer', Rajkovic told delegates.

'Try to convince kids to eat broccoli and it will take you probably 20 servings before they start to 'sort of' like it. Try

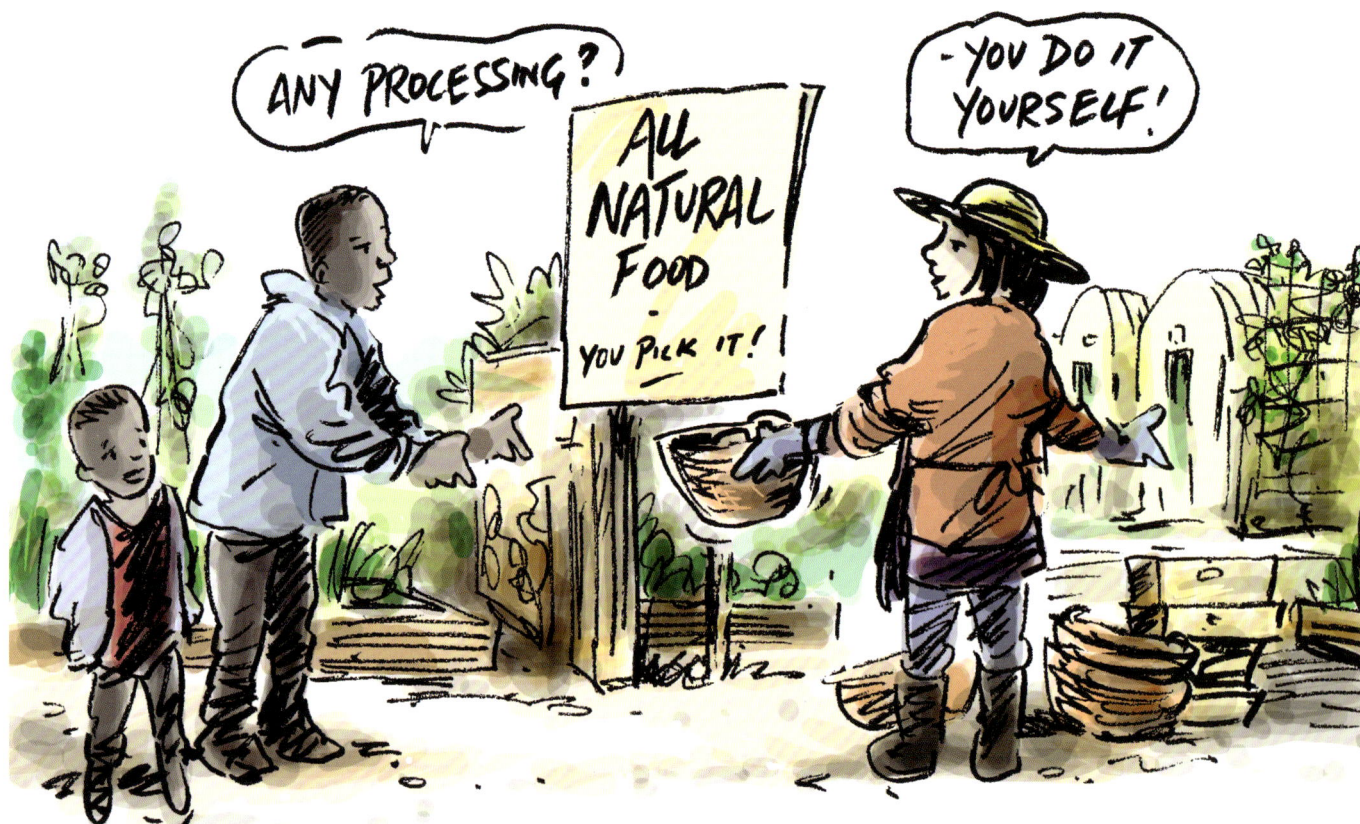

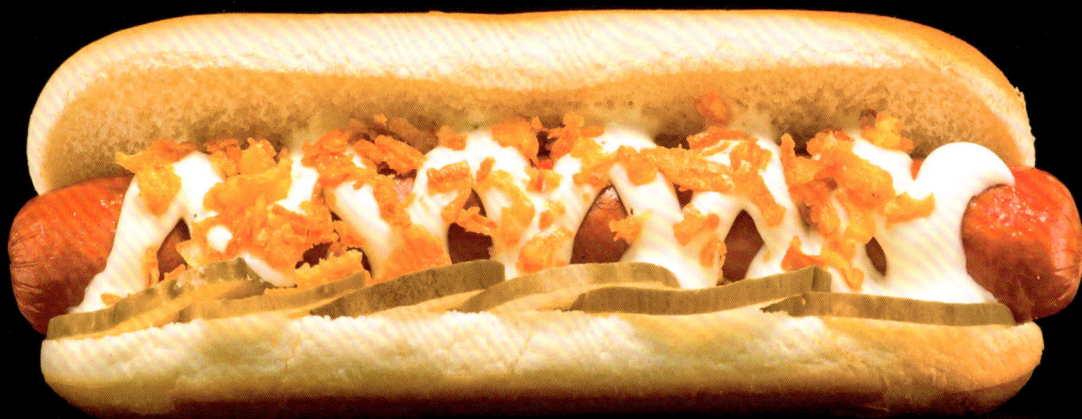

to give them ice cream, and it will take one or two times before they start liking it.

'So [in this instance], you could do something to help healthy broccoli consumption.'

Processed foods also align with the requirements of modern life, the food safety expert continued, referencing the importance of convenience in today's consumers. 'No processing and no 'smart additions' won't work for today's food choices.'

The business of food processing should also be perceived as a benefit. In Europe, the food industry employs close to 5 millon people and boasts a turnover of €1.2 trillion, which would be significantly impacted without the processing of food and food ingredients.

And finally, food processing enables innovation in the sector, said Rajkovic. 'The idea that you can modify food and create a new processes and products – and [in turn] bring something back to society – also turns society into engaged, employed personnel. And I think this is also very important to keep in mind.'

Processing done right

There are multiple instances where food processing has benefited human health. These examples, however, appear to receive less media attention in the 'processed foods' story.

During Rajkovic's presentation, he referred to the processing of grains – including sorting, trimming, cleaning, cooking, baking, frying and roasting – which can help reduce the amount of mycotoxin contamination.

Aflatoxins are one such kind of mycotoxin. Produced by certain moulds growing on agricultural crops, naturally occurring aflatoxins are classified as human carcinogens by the International Agency for Research on Cancer (IARC). 'Processing, therefore, takes something away from [the cereals] which we know is cancerogenic,' stressed Rajkovic.

Another example of food processing welcomed by health-conscious consumers – and in particular, those focused on calories and saturated fat intake – concerns low fat spread.

'One of the things in the modern world that we run away from is dense calorie intake,' explained the research professor. 'We want to use fat-reduced products so that we put lower amounts of dangerous fats in our body, such as saturated fats.'

One-hundred grams of conventional butter contains 80% fat and 737kcal. However, consumer demand for lower fat alternatives has prompted a 'healthier' response from manufacturers, Rajkovic told delegates.

The resulting low fat spread has half the calories of generic butter and just 35% fat. Of course, this 'healthy' alternative is processed. Emulsifiers are required due to the increased water activity in the product and additives are included to ensure long shelf-life and microbial food safety.

'There are good reasons to add stuff. Organic acids lower the pH and also work as an antimicrobial agent. Food preservatives and antioxidants inhibit microbial and chemical… spoilage. [And] fortifiers raise the nutrient levels in food,' we were told.

'If you don't do that, a lot of people in the world won't have enough Vitamin D or Vitamin C etc. So, there are things that sensibly need to be added.

'If you don't add, we are going to have a very fast growth of pathogens,' he said. 'The processing and additions of things are meaningful sometimes, if you know why we are doing it.'

A holistic approach

Rajkovic's professional opinion is that processed foods needn't be considered through a black and white lens. And moving forward, the consumer 'definitely' needs key elements from industry and government.

These include 'clear' information on the risks and benefits of processed foods. Consumers also require policy 'which is both protective and based on scientific evidence', but which Rajkovic stressed is 'not conservative' – so that it 'does not stop development'.

In such policies, respect for food, health, and environment should be present, as well as consideration for food waste. Climate change, obesity, and hunger should all be part of the equation, he continued.

The research professor also advocated for a 'holistic' approach to health. This should include lifestyle, exercise, sleep and stress. 'This is an important aspect.'

2 December 2020

8 tips for healthy eating during Ramadan

The most commonly consumed foods by Prophet Mohammed were milk, dates, lamb/mutton and oats. Healthy foods mentioned in the Holy Qur'an are fruit and vegetables, such as olives, onions, cucumber, figs, dates, grapes as well as pulses such as lentils. Complex carbohydrates are foods that will help release energy slowly during the long hours of fasting and are found in grains and seeds like barley, wheat, oats, millets, semolina, beans, lentils, wholemeal flour and basmati rice. Fibre-rich foods are also digested slowly and include bran, cereals, whole wheat, grains and seeds, potatoes with skin, vegetables such as green beans and almost all fruit, including apricots, prunes and figs. Foods to avoid are the heavily processed and fast-burning foods that contain refined carbohydrates such as sugar and white flour or fatty food like cakes, biscuits, chocolates and sweets. It may also be worth avoiding the caffeine content in drinks such as tea, coffee and cola (caffeine is a diuretic and stimulates faster water loss through urination).

Saher (sunrise) is the morning meal, served before dawn when the fast starts.

Iftar (sunset) is the evening snack when the fast is broken before dinner.

During Iftar, dates and juice are traditionally consumed. Include three dates and 4oz (120ml) of juice to help normalise possible low sugar (hypoglycaemia) and provide the much needed 'instant' energy along with hydration. *If you have diabetes, please consult with your healthcare provider for medication and diet.*

8 tips for healthy eating during Ramadan

1. Cut down on saturated fats, bake or grill foods instead of frying them, and if frying, decrease the amount of oil use. Try and measure the oil in a tablespoon instead of just pouring it from the bottle. All oils have the same fat and energy content. Oils such as rapeseed oil are a healthier choice, but still try to use as little as possible. Remember using 1 tablespoon of oil when cooking adds 120 kcal to your meal.

2. Choose lower fat and lean cuts of meat. Skin chicken and remove any visible fat before cooking. Having too much saturated fat can increase the amount of cholesterol in the blood, which increases the chance of developing heart disease. Try to avoid butter, ghee, lard and palm oil.

3. Eat lots of fruit and vegetables for better health. You should eat at least 5 portions of fruit and vegetables each day. Fruit and vegetables are high in vitamins and fibre as well as being low in fat.

4. Eat slowly and chew food well. Because you have not eaten all day, there will be a tendency to want to eat a large quantity of food quickly. Remember that it takes 20 minutes for your stomach to tell your brain that you are full – put small portions on your plate first.

5. Eating oily fish regularly can help reduce the risk of coronary heart disease and help protect your heart. Omega-3 fat is found in fresh and canned oily fish such as herring, mackerel, pilchard, sardines, salmon and fresh tuna. How does omega-3 protect the heart? It helps by making the heart to beat more regularly, reduces the stickiness of the blood, which makes it less likely to clot, and protects the arteries from damage. Aim for one serving of oily fish (high in omega-3) and one serving of white fish per week.

6. Walking in the evening for at least 30 minutes is an ideal activity. Walking will not only help your metabolism, but also help your mind stay clear. However, if you've eaten a big meal, blood needs to move to your digestive system rather than to your muscles, so a brisk walk straight after a heavy meal is not a good idea. Wait one to two hours after your meal before engaging in any strenuous activity. Best to keep your meals light.

7. Avoid too much caffeine. Caffeine is a diuretic and when consumed in large quantities can increase urine excretion and the body can lose valuable minerals such as salt and fluids that you need during the day.

8. Indigestion can be caused by over-eating or eating too many fried, fatty and spicy foods, or foods that produce gas. Fasting can also cause increased acidity, leading to the feeling of indigestion. To avoid indigestion, try not to over-eat. Be sure to drink plenty of water and include foods rich in fibre to neutralise acidity and promote a feeling of fullness.

7 October 2020

The alarming truth about ultra-processed foods – and why you should stop eating them

A fifth of Britons consume a diet that includes only a fifth of 'natural' foods, but there's more at risk than just weight gain.

By Xanthe Clay

What on earth is UPF? Ultra-processed foods, that's what, and this latest entry to our modern abbreviated lexicon is likely to be sticking around for a while – much like that bag of salted caramel pretzels (just one example of a UPF) on my hips.

The reason is that health professionals now want us to differentiate between simply 'processed' food and UPFs – foods that have been industrially altered to a high degree. Some are obvious, like a cheesy Wotsit, miraculously transformed from a grain of corn into a thumb-sized puff. But UPFs also include industrially produced bread, soy milk and other milk substitutes, breakfast cereals and baked beans.

That last inclusion in particular has got food manufacturers up in arms, as they point out that baked beans are a good source of protein and fibre and are relatively low in sugar and fat – although ingredients such as 'modified cornflour' and the hefty dose of artificial sweetener in the low-sugar versions are less edifying.

Processing is not necessarily a bad thing. Technically, processed foods are simply foods that have undergone a change – been processed, in fact – which may be simply to make them more digestible, or safer, or to preserve them. It can also, as Kate Halliwell, the chief scientific officer of the Food and Drink Federation recently pointed out in a letter to *The Telegraph*, be 'used to improve the nutritional value of food'.

So when wheat is ground and sifted to make white flour, that is a process. When it is fortified with calcium, iron, B vitamins (mandatory in the UK) and made into pasta, that is another two processes. And when it is dried, that is another process. When you boil it at home, that is yet another process. Some definitions include chewing – when you eat the pasta – and the harvesting of the grain as additional processes book-ending the journey from field to stomach.

Nonetheless, health experts are firm that UPFs generally are problematic, and certainly not something we should be eating every day. The definition of a UPF dates back to 2009 when the NOVA classification system (see below) was first developed by the University of São Paulo in Brazil. Foods are divided into four categories – unprocessed or minimally processed, culinary ingredients, processed, and ultra-processed – according to the way the food is used and how much it has been tinkered with during production.

It is not without controversy, however. Nutrition experts point out that some foods rated as highly nutritious, garnering an 'A' grade in the French Nutri-Score system (which is similar to the traffic light system seen on UK food packaging and current frontrunner to be adopted EU-wide) are labelled as ultra-processed (bad) by the NOVA classification. Others insist that Nutri-Score is over-simplistic, with no allowance for additives or industrial processing.

This is more than a storm in a Pot Noodle. While the anti-NOVA brigade have a point that no allowance is made in the classification for protein levels, for example, the evidence is mounting up that UPFs are behind the crisis that has seen obesity tripling worldwide since 1975. Here in the UK more than one in four adults are clinically obese, and in Europe only Turkey and Malta sit above us in the ranking.

Some readers will roll their eyes and say it is a matter of personal responsibility. And, yes, we probably do eat too much and don't exercise enough. No one is saying that eating a whole tube of Pringles (oh yes, I could) is healthier than a roast dinner, but seeing as both equate to about 1,000 calories, surely they will have the same effect on our waistline. A calorie is a calorie, right?

Increasingly, it seems not. In recent BBC programme *What Are We Feeding Our Kids?* Dr Chris Van Tulleken committed to a month of eating a diet of 80 per cent ultra-processed food, the same proportion of UPFs eaten by one in five Brits. The initial results were predictably depressing: he put on a stone and developed constipation, headaches and heartburn. He found his libido was reduced, he was eating more often, and was less satisfied by the processed food. But more significantly, scans showed that the activity in Van Tulleken's brain had changed in ways that mirror its response to substances like tobacco and alcohol, suggesting junk food is addictive.

As any scientist will tell you, one person eating a pile of junk food does not constitute proof that it is habit forming. But it is suggestive, and studies in America, including the Yale Food Addiction Scale, showed foods high in fat, salt, sugar and refined carbohydrates such as burgers, pizza, doughnuts, crisps and white bread can trigger dependence symptoms. There is also evidence that UPFs trigger an increase of the hunger hormone and decrease in the satiety hormone, making you want to eat more.

And think how easy junk food is. To eat, of course – that soft burger bun or the coating on chicken that crumbles and melts in the mouth. Chewing – unless it's gum – doesn't come into ultra processed food. The powerful flavours and pleasing textures have been tweaked by industry to get the exact levels of sugar, fat and salt to hit what they call 'the bliss point', making the product so irresistible we can't stop eating it. Sounds like courting addiction.

Unlike drugs, junk food is disarmingly easy to buy, handily packaged, and prominently displayed in the supermarket. It is simple to prepare, so convenient it seems churlish to pass it up. It is also cheap. According to *What Are We Feeding Our Kids?*, healthy foods such as vegetables, fruit and fresh fish cost more than double per hundred calories than less healthy convenience foods. The deal clincher for many of us is that they are part of our culture and childhood. If you, like me, were brought up on Angel Delight and fish fingers, then this is friendly, comforting home food.

So don't tell me this is about personal responsibility. As Prof Chris Millet points out to Van Tulleken, people 'haven't suddenly lost moral fibre over the last 20 or 30 years' as obesity has rocketed. What has changed in that time is the availability of junk food and the insidious way it has become the norm, weaselled its way into our fridges and food cupboards so that we no longer question what an 'olive oil spread' is actually made from or why pasta sauce has a shelf life of months.

There is no single solution to the obesity problem. But limiting the amount of ultra-processed food we eat is a good start. And if one thing delights me about the NOVA system, it is that it rewards real cooking. Sugar and fat are OK, if you are using them to cook something rather than buying a bag

of chips or a packet of biscuits. So we can still have treats provided they are homemade – which makes sense as then the majority of us will only get round to putting one on the table once a week, if that. Enough with the salted caramel pretzels, the Great British Pudding is back.

The NOVA food categories

Group 1: Unprocessed or minimally processed foods

Unprocessed foods are edible parts of plants (seeds, fruits, leaves, stems, roots) or of animals (including meat, fish, eggs and milk). Minimally processed foods include pasteurised milk, as well as food that has been simply dried, frozen or ground.

Group 2: Processed culinary ingredients

Includes oils, flour, butter, sugar and salt: foods not meant to be eaten alone.

Group 3: Processed foods

Most have two or three ingredients, and are made essentially by adding salt, oil, sugar or other substances from Group 2 to Group 1 foods. Includes canned fish, fruits in syrup, cheeses and freshly made breads. Ingredients may include preservatives and antioxidants.

Group 4: Ultra-processed foods

Includes many soft drinks, sweet or savoury packaged snacks, reconstituted meat and pre-prepared frozen dishes. Contains ingredients you wouldn't find in your kitchen, like casein and invert sugar. Additives may include colouring, flavour enhancers or emulsifiers. Manufacturing methods include processes you could not do at home, like hydrogenation and hydrolysation.

How to spot ultra-processed foods

♦ Download the Open Food Facts app, which has extensive listings so you can scan a barcode and check the NOVA group, Nutri-Score and Eco-Score (a French assessment of environmental impact) of over 1.8 million products worldwide. Check the list of ingredients. Does it include ones you can't visualise, like hydrolysed protein?

♦ Be wary of claims like 'made with wholegrains', 'high in iron' or 'no added sugar': while true in themselves, they may be giving a healthy whitewash to an essentially unhealthy, ultra processed food.

♦ Added 'natural flavourings' and 'natural colours' aren't naturally present in the food you are buying. Ask yourself why they are there: is it to cover up poor quality ingredients?

♦ Glitzy packaging and TV advertising don't necessarily mean a product is ultra processed, but be suspicious: UPFs have high profit margins which means heavy marketing makes good sense.

15 July 2021

In the news: will eating meat increase your risk of having a heart disease, diabetes or pneumonia?

Recent headlines claim that eating meat regularly could increase the risk of having up to 25 different diseases, including heart disease, diabetes and pneumonia. However, there are a few things to keep in mind when reading the study's conclusions.

The study behind the headlines

The recent news follows a new study that looks into the link between meat intake and the risk of 25 common conditions, other than cancer.

The study used data from adults (average age 55 years) registered in the UK Biobank.

Participants started by filling in a questionnaire (known as baseline dietary questionnaires) about their eating habits. They stated how often, how much and what type of meat they usually ate, differentiating between their consumption of red meat (unprocessed beef, unprocessed lamb/mutton and unprocessed pork), poultry and processed meat. There was no explanation of what was defined as processed meat. Some of the participants also completed other online questionnaires to see how their diet changed over time.

Researchers then followed up over a period of 8 years to assess the 25 most common causes (other than cancer) that led to participants being admitted to the hospital, by checking hospital admissions and mortality records.

Researchers concluded that those who ate red and processed meat and poultry regularly had a higher risk of developing several common diseases.

The results suggest that eating 70 grams of red and/or processed meat a day could increase the risk of heart disease, diabetes, pneumonia, diverticular disease and colon polyps roughly between 10-30%. More specifically, eating 50 grams of red meat a day was linked with an 8-21% higher risk of developing these five conditions while eating 20 grams of processed meat a day resulted in an 8-24% risk increase.

More so, eating 30 grams of poultry a day was linked with a higher risk of diabetes and different digestive diseases, such as reflux disease and irritation/inflammation of the stomach and the large bowel.

What to keep in mind when reading the study's conclusions?

Observational studies can't prove direct cause and effect.

The study has taken into account multiple health and lifestyle factors such as age, ethnicity, overall diet, body mass index (BMI) and physical activity, that could potentially influence the health outcomes considered. However, the researchers caution that even so, it's not entirely possible to ensure that such factors had no impact on the final results.

Estimates of meat intake may be inaccurate.

While food frequency questionnaires are one of the best methods available to assess dietary intake, they still have limitations. For example, estimates of the frequency, amount and type of meat eaten (such as what an individual considers to be processed meat) may be subjective and vary between participants. Also, the analysis didn't assess relevant dietary details such as how meat was prepared (if it was a lean or a fatty cut) or cooked (whether it was grilled or fried, for example).

Meat consumption also has dietary benefits, which need to be considered when reducing intake.

Lean unprocessed red and white meat are good sources of protein and various other nutrients, such as iron, zinc and vitamin B12. Notably, the study found that the intake of both red meat and poultry was linked with a lower risk of anaemia from iron deficiency. When considering decreasing meat intake to reduce any of the potential risks identified, it's important to add enough plant-based sources of these nutrients to meet our needs.

The study only considered a specific group of UK participants and may not be representative of other populations.

This was a large study, but it included mostly middle-aged adults (average age 55 years) of white ethnicity (90% of participants) from the UK. Other populations and ethnic groups, with different health, lifestyle and genetic characteristics may have a different disease risk.

What do authorities say?

♦ National advice on how much red meat people should eat regularly varies, ranging from a maximum recommended intake of 70g a day (350g per week) in the UK to 500g a week in Scandinavian countries.[2]

♦ In general, most countries recommend choosing lean meats removed of any visible fat, over red meat. Plus, most encourage limiting the consumption of processed meat within a weekly or a daily maximum, when not to avoid it completely.[2] You can learn how these recommendations translate to food portions by consulting your national dietary guidelines.

♦ The World Health Organization (WHO) recognises that diets high in processed and/or red meats can increase the risk of some types of cancers.[3] In turn, the Mediterranean diet – characterised by low consumption of meat (particularly red meat) and saturated fat and by being high in plant-based sources of protein, such as legumes – has been found to reduce the risk of adverse health outcomes such as cardiovascular disease.[4]

♦ If you wish to reduce or cut meat and/or animal products from your diet, consider consulting a professional or registered nutritionist to get professional advice on how to make it in a healthy way.

References

2. EU Joint Research Centre. Health Promotion & Disease Prevention – Food-based Dietary Guidelines in Europe. Accessed on 6 Mar. 2021
3. World Health Organisation (WHO) (2015). Healthy Diet Factsheet No 394. Accessed on 6 Mar. 2021
4. World Health Organisation (WHO) (2015). Cancer: Carcinogenicity of the consumption of red meat and processed meat. Accessed on 6 Mar. 2021

10 March 2021

www.eufic.org

Reducing the risk of type 2 diabetes

This article is aimed at people who do not have a diagnosis of type 2 diabetes but would like to learn more about how they can reduce their risk of developing this condition.

Key messages

♦ **Type 1 and type 2 diabetes occur when sugar in the blood cannot be used properly, and this can cause serious health complications.**

♦ **About 90% of people with diabetes have type 2 diabetes.**

♦ **Type 2 diabetes is strongly linked with overweight and obesity and can be prevented.**

♦ **Although there are several risk factors for type 2 diabetes that are beyond control, eating a healthy, varied diet, being physically active and losing weight (if necessary) can greatly help to reduce the risk of developing this condition.**

♦ Type 2 diabetes tends to be diagnosed in people aged over 40 years. However, increasingly, the symptoms are being seen in younger adults and even children.

♦ Type 2 diabetes is strongly linked with overweight and obesity, although not all people with type 2 diabetes are overweight or obese.

♦ This condition can generally be treated by making lifestyle changes, such as eating a healthy, varied diet and doing regular physical activity. Sometimes oral medication (such as metformin) and/or insulin are also needed.

About 10% of people with diabetes have **type 1 diabetes.**

♦ This condition cannot be prevented and occurs when cells in the pancreas that produce insulin have been

What is diabetes?

In the UK, it is estimated that 3.8 million people aged over 16 years have been diagnosed with diabetes and nearly 1 million are unaware that they have the condition. Diabetes occurs when the body cannot use sugar properly. As a result, there can be high levels of sugar in the blood, if the condition is not controlled.

People with diabetes can lead a full and active life. However, if blood sugar levels are uncontrolled, it can cause several serious health problems over time involving the eyes, heart, kidneys, feet and nerves. Serious short-term complications also exist for people who depend on insulin to control their diabetes. This includes diabetic ketoacidosis (when blood sugar levels are consistently very high) and hypoglycaemia (when blood sugar levels are too low).

It is especially important for those diagnosed with diabetes to control their blood sugar levels and their blood pressure, to eat a healthy diet, be physically active and to lose weight if necessary.

There are two main types of diabetes:

About 90% of people with diabetes have **type 2 diabetes.**

♦ This condition occurs when the body either cannot produce enough insulin (the hormone needed to move sugar from the blood into the body's cells) or the insulin the body produces is not used properly (known as insulin resistance), leading to sugar build up in the blood.

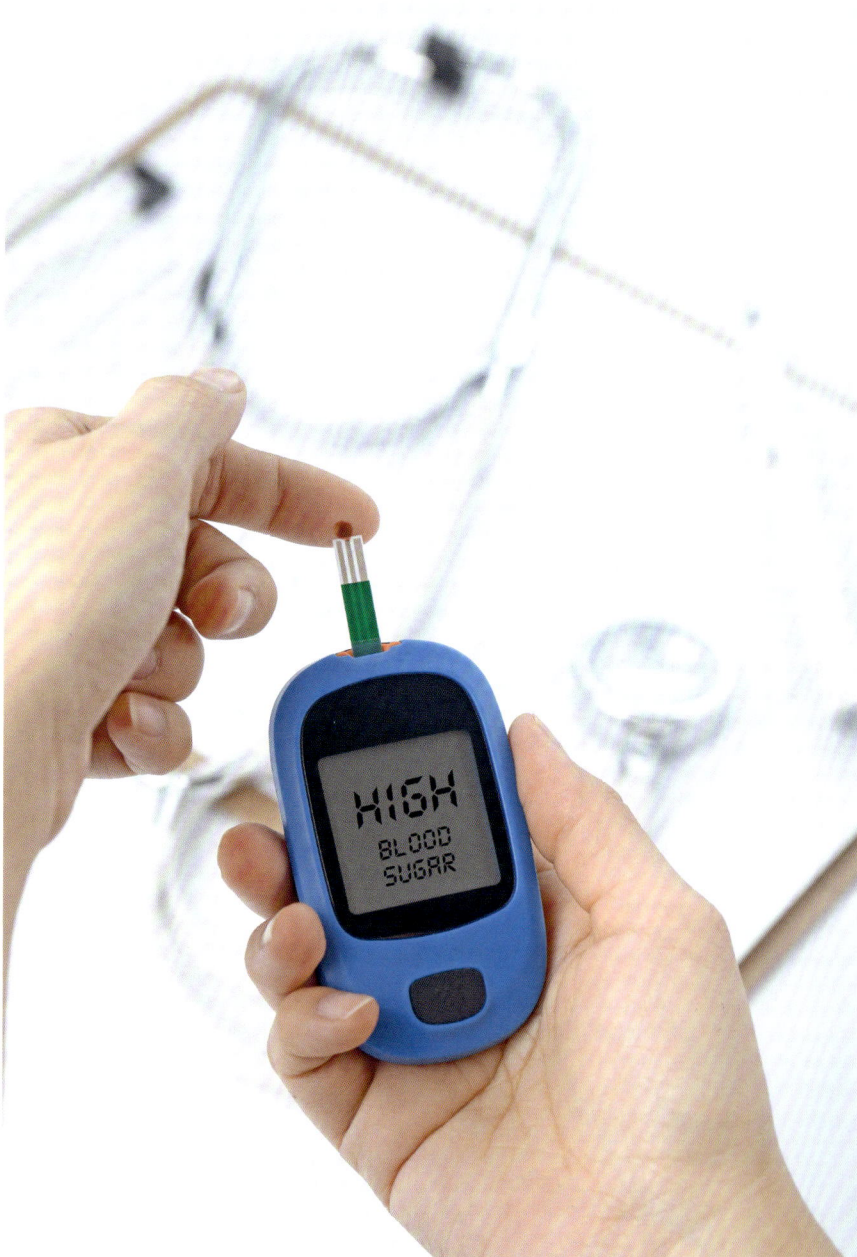

destroyed by the immune system.

- In type 1 diabetes there is no insulin and so sugar stays in the blood.
- This means that people with type 1 diabetes need to take insulin (either with an injection or an insulin pump) to help the body use sugar properly and control blood sugar levels.
- Nobody fully understands why the insulin-producing cells in the pancreas become damaged, but it may be triggered by a viral or other infection.

What are the risk factors for type 2 diabetes?

There are certain risk factors that can increase the likelihood of developing type 2 diabetes. You cannot change all of them, but you can make some changes to your lifestyle that will help to reduce your risk.

Your weight

Around 90% of people diagnosed with type 2 diabetes are overweight or obese. The more overweight you are the greater your risk, with obese people being seven times more likely to develop type 2 diabetes than people with a healthy bodyweight. To find out if you are overweight ask your GP to measure your BMI (body mass index) - a healthy BMI is 18.5-25 kg/m2. A healthy, varied diet and regular exercise can help you lose weight gradually and help keep it off.

Your waist

Women – if your waist measures 80cm or more you have an increased risk of developing type 2 diabetes; the risk is very high if it is more than 88cm.

Men – if your waist measures 94cm or more you have an increased risk of developing type 2 diabetes; if you are male with South Asian background the measurement is 90cm or more; the risk is very high if it is more than 102cm.

Your age

You are at increased risk of type 2 diabetes if you are over 40 years of age; if your background is Black African, Chinese, South Asian or African-Caribbean, you are at increased risk if you are over 25 years of age. The risk continues to increase with age. Of course, you cannot change your age but you can work on the other risk factors to reduce your risk.

Your family history

You cannot change your family history either but having type 2 diabetes in the family increases your risk. The closer the relative is, the greater the risk. Tell your GP whether anyone in your family has type 2 diabetes. If you know that type 2 diabetes runs in your family, make sure that you are doing all you can to reduce your risk in other ways.

Your ethnicity

Some ethnic groups have higher risk of type 2 diabetes than others and are likely to be affected at an earlier age (see 'Your age' section above). If you have an African-Caribbean or South Asian background and live in the UK, then you are at least three times more likely to have type 2 diabetes than the White population and it is particularly important for you to make sure that you maintain a healthy bodyweight.

Lifestyle factors

Several lifestyle factors, some of which are linked to overweight and obesity, have been associated with an increased risk of developing type 2 diabetes. These include smoking, being sedentary and eating an unhealthy diet.

Other factors

You may also have an increased risk of having type 2 diabetes if you:

- have high blood pressure or if you've had a heart attack or a stroke
- are a woman with a history of polycystic ovary syndrome, gestational diabetes (a temporary type of diabetes during pregnancy) or have given birth to a large baby
- have been told you have impaired glucose tolerance or metabolic syndrome.

Multiple risk factors

The more risk factors that apply to you, the greater the risk of developing type 2 diabetes.

How can I reduce the risk of developing type 2 diabetes?

Eating a healthy, varied diet, being physically active and losing weight (if necessary) can reduce your risk of type 2 diabetes.

Become more active

Try to be physically active and maintain a healthy bodyweight (BMI 18.5-25 kg/m2) to reduce your risk of type 2 diabetes. It is recommended that adults choose activities that include aerobic and strength exercises. The recommended minimum amount of physical activity for adults per week is 150 minutes of moderate level aerobic activity (this should raise your heart rate and make you breathe faster and feel warmer) or 75 minutes of vigorous aerobic activity (this should make you breathe hard and fast) (or a mix of the two types of aerobic activity). Plus strength exercises (such as yoga, exercises like sit ups or press ups or heavy gardening like digging) on two or more days of the week.

But don't worry - you do not have to join a gym! Walking, dancing, swimming, gardening, golf, bowling and cycling are all activities that count towards physical activity. Activity can also be spread out through the day so you can make small changes to your lifestyle, which can add up to a lot more activity. For example, use the stairs instead of taking the lift, leave the car at home for small trips, or get off the bus one or two stops earlier. Even housework can count! These are all achievable ways to incorporate activity into your daily routine.

Eat a healthy, varied diet

Making healthy food choices and cutting down on the amount of energy (calories) you consume can help achieve a healthy bodyweight and maintain weight loss (if needed) and reduce your risk of developing type 2 diabetes. Calorie and portion size control is very important for those wishing to lose weight.

In the UK it is recommend that a healthy, varied diet is based on starchy foods and plenty of fruit and vegetables, and is low in saturated fat, sugar and salt. These recommendations are based on the latest evidence and apply to the general population. For more information see our pages on a healthy and sustainable diet.

If you have a diagnosis of diabetes, foods containing starchy carbohydrates remain an important part of a healthy, varied diet. However, as these foods affect blood sugar levels, it is recommended that you talk with your diabetes healthcare team about the best type and amount to incorporate into your diet.

The following recommendations will help you eat a healthy, varied diet:

♦ Try to eat meals at regular times throughout the day.

♦ Base meals on starchy foods, such as potatoes, rice, pasta, bread and breakfast cereals, choosing wholegrain or higher fibre versions where possible.

♦ Just over a third of the food we eat each day should be fruit and vegetables. Aim for at least five portions a day and try to eat a variety; green leafy vegetables in particular are associated with reduced risk of type 2 diabetes.

♦ Foods high in saturated fat and sugars, such as chocolate, cakes, biscuits, full-sugar soft drinks, butter and ice-cream are not needed in the diet and so, if included, should only be eaten infrequently and in small amounts.

♦ Choose beans, pulses and other vegetable sources of protein (like tofu), lean meat, poultry and fish, instead of fatty meat or processed meat products.

♦ Choose low-fat and low-sugar dairy foods, such as skimmed or semi-skimmed milk and low-fat, unsweetened yogurt.

♦ Use unsaturated oils, such as vegetable, rapeseed and olive oils, in cooking but only in small amounts. Swap butter for lower fat spreads.

♦ Where possible, use cooking methods that reduce the amount of fat in your dishes (such as grilling meat and fish instead of frying and have a boiled or poached egg instead of fried).

♦ Choose products lower in salt and use less salt in cooking.

♦ If you drink alcohol, do so in moderation - no more than 14 units per week for both men and women.

♦ Keep hydrated, try to drink 6-8 glasses of fluid a day. Swap sugary soft drinks for those without sugar, such as water, tea, coffee and diet drinks.

2021

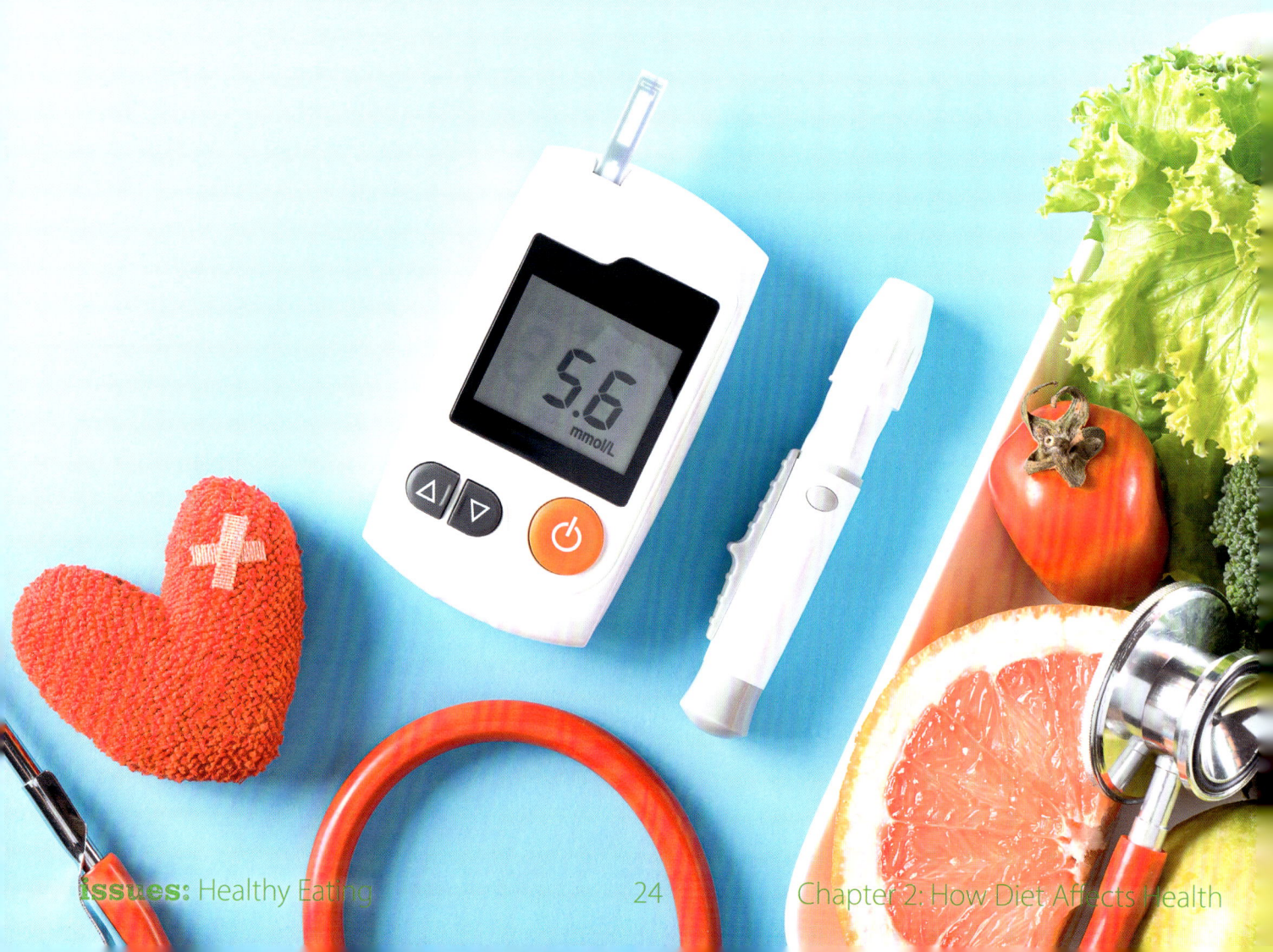

Rise in UK child obesity

Digital data collected by the NHS show that there has been an increase in childhood obesity over the pandemic.

By Charlotte Hurst

Although obesity has risen for all changes, the most worrying age group is those within their last year of primary school. Here, general rates have risen from 21% to 25%. However, in poorer areas, rates have increased by twice the amount.

Dr Max Davie of Paediatrics and Child Health discusses how 'lockdown may have been a key factor, [but] we mustn't assume that this year's results are an aberration since there may have been other factors'.

Other potential factors include rises in poverty and mental health issues.

When regarding how to address this concerning issue, Carolin Cemy, of the Obesity Health Alliance, states 'We need to break the junk-food cycle to improve children's obesity'.

However, this will most likely only provide a short term fix, as it glosses over the root causes of the problem.

Estimate of child obesity jumps during covid

Proportion of **overweight** and **obese** children in their final year of primary school in England

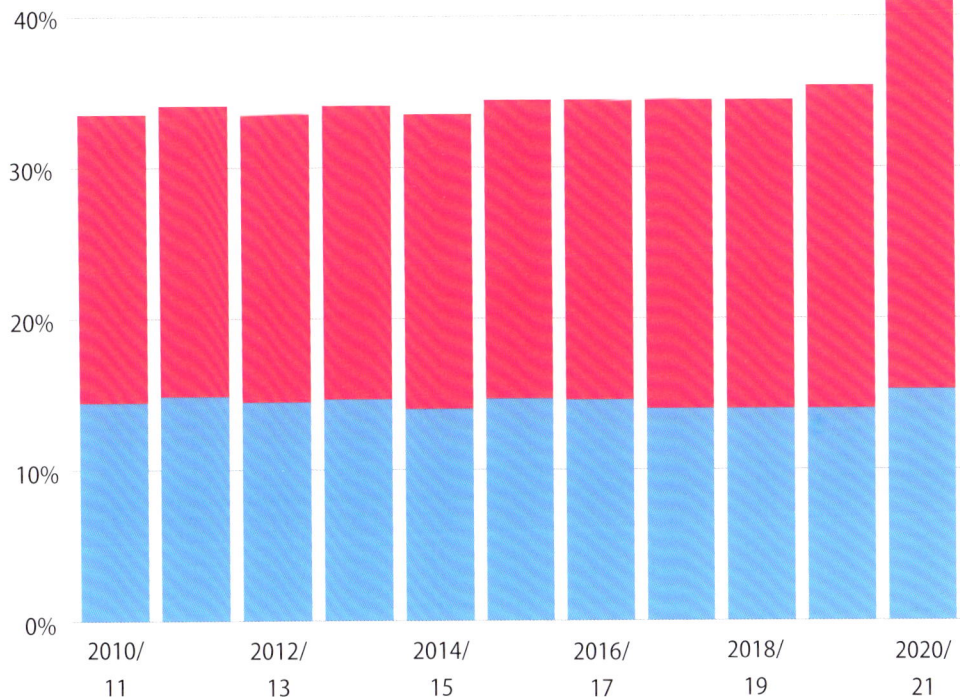

2020/21 estimate based on measurements from 24% of children rather than entire school year

Source: NHS Digital, National Child Measurement Programme in England

The annual *Broken Plate* report found that the average cost of healthy food in 2019 was around £7.68. This is much higher than the £2.48 cost of less healthy food with the same caloric intake.

Therefore, advocating for healthier foods will make little difference for those who cannot afford it, even if they want to change their diets.

A long term solution is harder to come to than perceived. This is due to so many factors contributing to the problem.

One starting point, however, would be directly acknowledging the roles that social and economic factors play in health problems.

Furthermore, actions need to be taken in all areas of Government, as the issue has grown to such a scale it has become too large for the Department of Health and Social Care to tackle alone.

The Government's proposed scheme to 'level up' may also provide some solution to child obesity. If it tackles the growing inequality gap within UK society, families may have a larger disposable income to afford the healthy food that contributes to good health.

Higher wages may also help to achieve this, as it may prevent parents from working long hours as they may now earn more. This would give them time to prepare healthy meals.

However, until the factors of child obesity are addressed, the issue will grow.

Currently, there are 36,000 nursing vacancies within the NHS, creating a waiting list of around 6,000,000. The high waiting list means that many children won't get the treatment they require.

This could potentially even result in a lower quality of education that they receive as they may be spending more time off school ill than learning.

Therefore, the issue of child obesity is more concerning than most perceive it to be.

24 November 2021

British consumers complicit in forty-year 'healthy eating' failure, new study suggests

'Healthy eating' campaigns have largely failed in Britain for the last four decades because consumers have adapted confusing advice, and incorporated fast and convenience foods into self-defined 'balanced' lifestyles, a new study argues.

Supermarkets and food manufacturers have been excessively blamed for Britain's unhealthy eating habits since the 1980s, according to Cambridge historian Dr Katrina-Louise Moseley.

In an article published in *Contemporary British History*, Moseley argues that far from being passive victims of manipulation in this period, consumers were 'complicit' in long-term behavioural shifts, proactively selecting, rejecting and sweetening advice from the government, the food industry and the media to fit their circumstances and to satisfy their appetites.

Rather than seeking to cast blame, Moseley asserts that we should think more carefully about how people rationalise their eating behaviours and interpret advice about food. Speaking ahead of a public event entitled 'Food on the Move' (9 July 2021), Moseley added that this is particularly relevant in the context of the COVID-19 pandemic, which has had a dramatic impact on eating behaviours.

'Food is a powerful coping mechanism in times of emotional distress, so it isn't surprising that people have been buying extra packets of their favourite snack or eating more takeaways. I'm interested in the psychology of consumption and getting away from moralising language around food, which can be damaging', Moseley said. As part of the event, hosted by the University of Warwick, Moseley invites readers to complete an anonymous survey (closes 9 July 2021) to reflect on how their own food practices have changed during the pandemic.

In her article, Moseley contrasts the success of Britain's anti-smoking campaign, which transformed attitudes to tobacco in the 1960s and 70s, with the failure of the 'healthy eating' campaign to counteract rising levels of obesity from the late 1980s onwards.

Moseley said: 'The state faced a really difficult task. "Don't smoke" was a clear-cut message but you can't tell people not to eat. Food can't be rejected outright, it has to remain a part of everyday life, and that makes it so much more complicated. We're still really struggling with this today.'

The historian makes fresh use of consumer interviews and surveys conducted in England and Wales in the 1980s and 90s. These include a Mass Observation directive questionnaire on 'Food and Drink' completed in 1982; interviews and participant observations gathered from 1992–96 in response to the 1992 *Health of the Nation* report; and a collection of life history interviews undertaken with a sample of older people in 2017–18.

Moseley argues that a major problem facing Britain's 'healthy eating' campaign has been its reliance, often unavoidable, on malleable language. Words like 'balance' and 'moderation' left themselves open to subjective interpretation. Moseley

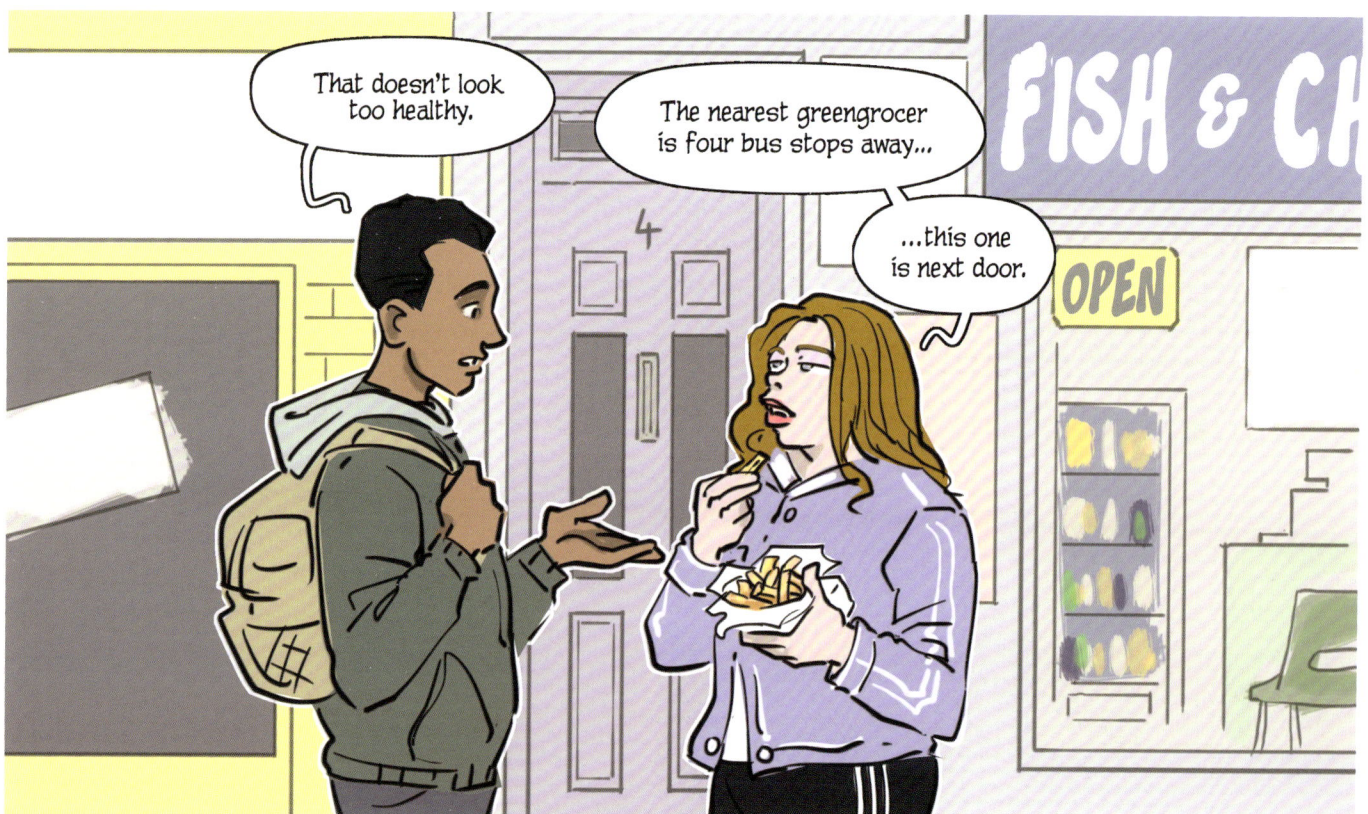

said: 'These records reveal all kinds of people, not just the less affluent, leaning towards convenience foods while still trying to define their lifestyles as healthy.'

Looking at the 1982 questionnaire records, Moseley found that attitudes to convenience foods were 'shot through with contradictions'. Speaking for herself and her husband, one female respondent claimed, 'neither of us can bear ready-made frozen dinners' – but she made 'an exception for certain things from Marks & Spencer – their frozen cod in parsley sauce is palatable and their cauliflower cheese makes me a quick solo meal if Neil is out for the evening.'

Moseley said: 'For health enthusiasts and cynics alike, official information about food didn't always feel correct. Consumers continued to assert that foods had different effects on different individuals, that one could be overweight whilst leading a healthy lifestyle, and that – in the midst of a dizzying array of information, self-evaluation was key.'

The study describes how supermarkets and food manufacturers seized on the idea of 'healthy eating' in the 1980s in response to new nutritional guidelines being issued. In 1984, Heinz began a 25-year-programme to reduce salt and sugar in its products; and in 1986 Mars produced a pamphlet entitled 'Confectionary in a Healthy Diet'. Meanwhile Tesco and Sainsbury's turned their attention to nutritional labelling.

> ## "These records reveal all kinds of people ... leaning towards convenience foods while still trying to define their lifestyles as healthy"
>
> – Katrina-Louise Moseley

Moseley said: 'We underestimate what a pivotal role the convenience foods sector played in producing and disseminating knowledge about 'healthy eating' in this period. Sometimes, as with Findus' calorie-controlled ready meals, it was the food industry rather than politicians or doctors that gave people usable, workable public health messages. But increasingly people came to view big food companies, government and public health experts as one and the same: a mysterious force manipulating consumer behaviour.'

Testimonies collected in the 1980s and 90s emphasise that new jargon baffled many consumers. Puzzling over the term 'polyunsaturated margarine', one respondent to the 1980s questionnaire said: 'I understand that poly means many and unsaturated means not chock full of something, so what is margarine poly unsaturated with or not with?' In 1985, a market research study of nearly 1,500 consumers in England and Wales found that 43% were uncertain whether saturated or polyunsaturated fat was better for them.

Moseley said: 'Terms like "E-numbers" and "saturated fats" entered public discourse but that didn't mean that everyone understood or accepted health advice, let alone changed their behaviours. Naturally, people embraced foods that made their lives easier and their mealtimes tastier, often using the language of "moderation" to justify the consumption of highly processed, time-saving foods.'

The study examines the rise of scepticism as consumers felt overloaded with confusing, contradictory and unreliable 'healthy eating' messages. The 1992–96 interviews reveal that consumers became increasingly committed to using their 'common sense' when thinking about food. Moseley said: 'Consumers didn't respond as authorities hoped they would, but they weren't irrational or lacking in judgement. People subscribed to their own, highly personalized logics.'

One 1992–96 interviewee said: 'some days you just want mashed potatoes and I'm not going to feel bad about that because with the rest of my life… it's balanced'. Interviewees also sought reassurance from their childhood eating habits or those of older relatives, saying things like: 'Nan lived to a good old age' or 'it didn't seem to do us much harm at the time'.

Testimonies from the 1990s also reveal the emergence of a new language linking food and feeling. One woman defined healthy eating as 'that difference between… getting a good feeling from what you eat and getting this sort of not very nice feeling'. 'Cheese especially' made another young woman feel 'so ugh – you know it makes me feel so fat and just weighs me down'. She added that she felt 'much healthier and brighter' if she avoided it.

Moseley said: 'The idea that different foods might cause individuals to feel a certain way in their bodies prefigured a major shift towards self-diagnosed food intolerances in the early twenty-first century.'

The study accepts that some positive health trends did come about in the late 20th century but points out that consumers favoured easier quick-fixes like switching to brown bread and semi-skimmed milk, over sweeping dietary transformations.

Moseley said: 'Medical researchers remain very worried about public scepticism, but their studies tend to lack historical context. Thinking about the history of trust and cynicism alongside developments in public health can help us understand and reconstruct the bigger picture.'

Reflecting on Britain's food culture today, Moseley points out that economic, social and geographic constraints on 'healthy' choices lack public visibility: factors like deprivation, time poverty, and mental illness delimit the choices that consumers feel able to make. She said: 'Too often, health education campaigns promote 'informed' decision making around food, as if social and economic disparities do not exist. Food has long been a site of inequality in Britain, and unfortunately it remains so today.'

1 July 2021

Reference

K Moseley, 'From Beveridge Britain to Birds Eye Britain: Shaping knowledge about "healthy eating" in the mid-to-late twentieth-century', Contemporary British History (2021). DOI: 10.1080/13619462.2021.1915141

Nutrition in adolescence: multiple challenges, lifelong consequences and the foundation for adult health

An article from *The Conversation*.

THE CONVERSATION

By Jo-Anna B. Baxter, Postdoctoral Research Fellow, Department of Nutritional Sciences, University of Toronto

Around the world, there are an estimated 1.2 billion adolescents between 10 and 19 years old. Although adolescence lies between childhood and adulthood, adolescents are neither big children, nor little adults. They have increased food requirements to support their rapid physical growth and maturation.

The steep increase in issues such as anaemia, overweight and obesity in this age group puts nutritional issues among the greatest immediate threats to adolescent health. Exposure to healthy nutrition from adolescence — ranging from actual food consumption to the food environment — can set the stage for a healthy life ahead and good dietary habits.

The combined factors that shape diet can include personal factors, such as taste preferences and knowledge of healthy foods; social influences like friends, families and co-workers; and physical surroundings, including stores and advertising.

However, poverty and socio-economic inequalities remain important barriers to accessing diverse and nutritious foods. Supporting adolescents' health and well-being is necessary to ensure their healthy development, but also offers lifelong and intergenerational benefits.

From a lifelong perspective, healthy eating behaviours adopted during adolescence, such as how much and what you eat, are more likely to continue into adulthood. Intergenerationally, things like adolescent pregnancy can negatively affect a girl's growth, and can also impact fetal growth and development.

Forms of malnutrition in adolescents

Adolescents face forms of malnutrition on both ends of the spectrum, from being underweight and having micronutrient deficiencies, to being overweight and obesity.

On the undernutrition side, an estimated one in four adolescents experience anaemia, a condition where someone does not have enough healthy red blood cells to carry adequate oxygen to their body's tissues. Linked to limited intake of required vitamins and minerals or malabsorption from the gut, anaemia can complicate growth and development.

Anaemia can also decrease productivity, which is particularly important considering most adolescents go to school and/or work. The number of adolescents who experience undernutrition is disproportionately higher in low- and middle-income countries.

From an over-nutrition perspective, one in five adolescents is overweight or obese, and the proportion is increasing worldwide. These conditions are associated with a greater risk of developing a disease such as diabetes or cancer later in life, as well as chronic health issues such as hypertension.

Making nutritious food choices

Eating a balanced and diverse diet is key to meeting nutritional needs. Making good food choices is complicated by adolescents' affinity for unhealthy foods, such as high-energy and ultra-processed foods like sugar-sweetened drinks and fast food. Compared to children, they have a greater say in what they eat, when and where they eat it, and can be increasingly influenced by social pressures.

Food environments are shaped by food availability, affordability, promotion, quality and safety. They impact food choices and are an important factor in what adolescents eat. Adolescents can face multiple food environments daily between the different settings they encounter such as home, school and workplace.

Food environments can be classified into three categories:

♦ **Traditional:** Limited food availability and accessibility, adolescent food autonomy is restricted.

♦ **Mixed:** Greater food availability and affordability, food autonomy is increased, role for social significance of food and advertising.

♦ **Modern:** No concerns about food access, food autonomy is common, influenced by peers and advertising.

Poverty's effect on healthy food consumption

In resource-limited settings, found in both high- and low-income countries, poverty is a key factor driving nutritional inequalities — particularly micronutrient deficiencies. With the COVID-19 pandemic, economically vulnerable households worldwide have experienced increased food challenges and food insecurity. This presents yet another challenge to adolescent nutrition.

With colleagues in Pakistan, my research looked at social determinants of nutrition among late adolescent girls. One way we did this was using a diet scoring tool to assess the diversity of the food they ate. We found that the adolescent girls ate micronutrient-poor foods most of the time, and they commonly had highly sweetened tea, desserts and fried snacks.

We investigated the roles of different factors thought to affect adolescent nutrition, including education level, food insecurity, self-efficacy and decision-making autonomy. We

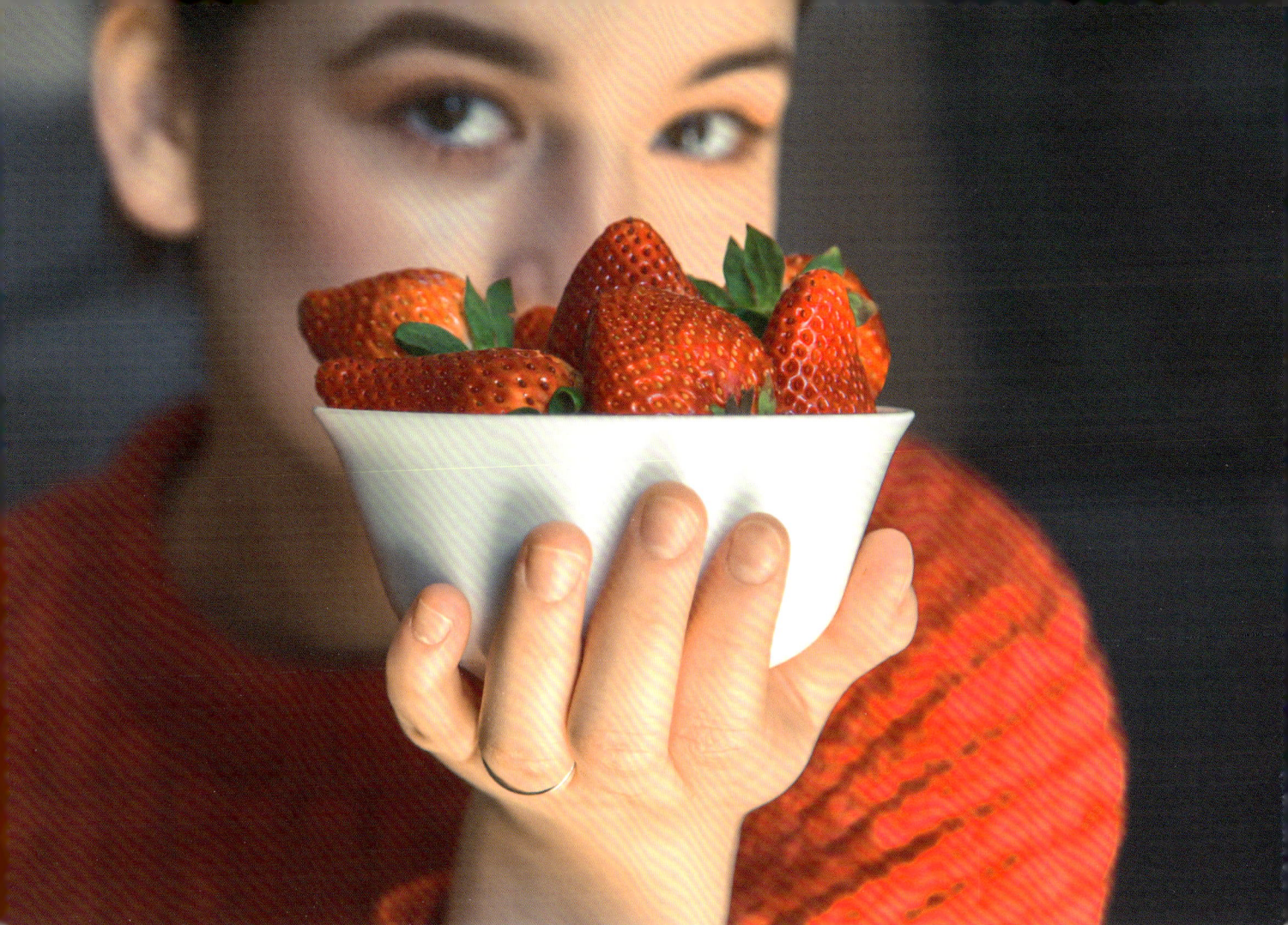

found poverty was the most important factor predicting a limited diet. In this traditional food environment, addressing adolescent girls' dietary quality will require two components:

1. Strategies to reduce poverty to deal with the resource constraints that prevented them from accessing diverse and nutritious foods. These include social safety net programs such as cash transfers.

2. Micronutrient intake strategies such as supplements and fortified foods.

Interventions to improve adolescent nutrition

The World Health Organization recognizes several evidence-informed interventions to improve nutrition during adolescence. These range from education to supplements, and vary depending on the setting, context and type of malnutrition.

For example, a nutrition intervention targeting adolescents in Canada would look different from one in Pakistan. However, interventions within either Canada or Pakistan could also differ, depending on geography (urban or rural) and resources. In settings with socio-economic barriers such as income and education, these must be addressed; intervening at the individual level alone does not get at the root cause of malnutrition.

A recent international study looked at the interventions in different countries to improve adolescents' food and nutrition environments and increase their ability to make choices about their nutrition. It showed a need for more data and research, and saw a role for engaging adolescents to generate solutions. But the greatest reach may come from establishing collaborations across multiple sectors. This means extending beyond the usual players in health and nutrition to engage those in education, food production and marketing (including social media), and agriculture.

Today's adolescents face multiple threats to their nutrition. Accessing a healthy and safe diet is a basic need, yet nutritional inequalities are on the rise between and within countries. Addressing underlying inequalities and providing appropriate nutrition interventions for adolescents offer a long-term positive impact on their lives.

8 February 2022

Healthier diets 'three times as expensive', claims Food Foundation report

Foods that are high in sugar fat are only 40% of the cost of fruit & vegetables per each 1,000 calories.

By Maria Gonclaves

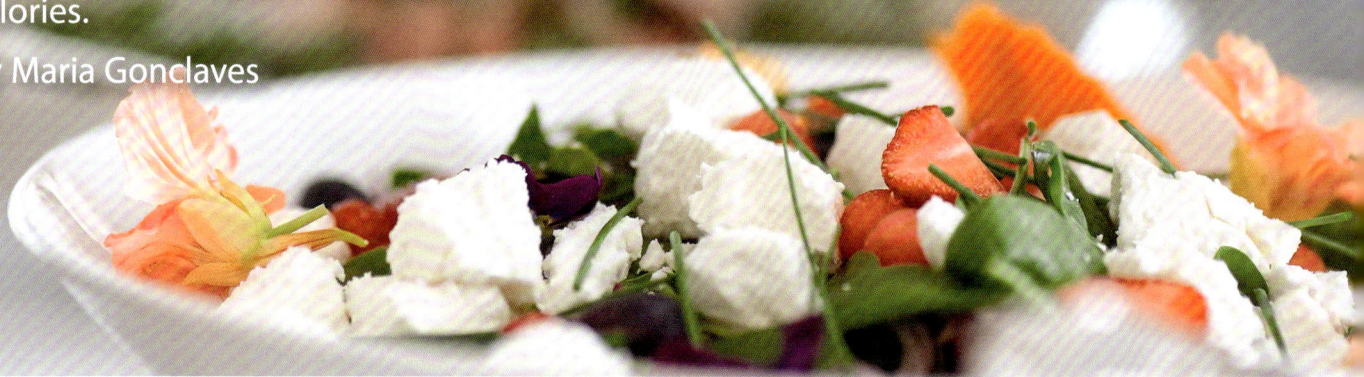

According to the *Broken Plate Report*, foods that are high in sugar and fat are cheaper than healthier foods

Healthier foods are currently nearly three times as expensive as their less healthy counterparts, according to a new report from the Food Foundation.

The annual *Broken Plate Report* said dietary inequality, obesity levels, and 'critically low levels' of healthy food consumption contributed to a 'broken' current food system in the UK.

According to the study, foods that are high in sugar and fat are only 40% of the cost of fruit & vegetables per each 1,000 calories.

In addition, the poorest fifth of the country's households would need to spend 40% of their income on healthier food to be able to meet the government's Eatwell Guide costs, compared with 5% for the wealthiest fifth.

'For people with less money available it is likely to be harder to afford and therefore eat a varied and healthy diet rich in fruit & vegetables,' said Dr Kate Ellis of the University of Cambridge. 'This leaves people reliant on less healthy, energy-dense foods to make up the majority of their diet. While these price differences remain, it will be hard to tackle dietary inequalities in the UK.'

The survey also claimed one third of places to buy food in communities with lower incomes are fast food outlets, compared to one fifth in 'least deprived' local authorities. Fast food consumption is linked to chronic diseases such as obesity and diabetes.

According to the report, over half of the children born in 2021 will experience diet-related diseases by the time they are 65 years old. Children in the 'most deprived decile' were 10 times more likely to develop severe obesity by the age of 11 than those in the 'least deprived decile'.

'Some of this year's findings are quite shocking and sets us all a big challenge for this year ahead, particularly those who work to change public policy and industry ambition for the benefit of consumers,' said Food Foundation chair of trustees Laura Sandys.

The annual study showed that advertising spend on fruit & veg decreased in 2020 from the year before, corresponding to only 2.5% of the total food and soft drink advertising spend. It said that 92% of cereals and 96% of yoghurts marketed for children contained 'high or medium' levels of sugar.

'Our new Secretary of State for Health & Social Care must confront the food companies promoting and profiting from unhealthy processed food which, as we know, can lead to obesity and the worse outcomes from Covid-19,' said Katharine Jenner, campaign director at Action on Sugar.

Meanwhile, the costs of vegetarian and plant-based meals generally dropped since last year's survey, with 22% of ready meals being vegetarian or plant-based.

Eating Better executive director Simon Billing said that while there had been some progress on upping vegetable content in ready meals, there was still 'much more work to do' to make healthier and sustainable food choices affordable for the general population.

The *Broken Plate Report*, which was funded by the Nuffield Foundation, was released ahead of the Henry Dimbleby-led National Food Strategy review. The NFS is expected to include strict recommendations to government to improve the food sector across all levels.

'There has never been a more opportune time for the government and businesses to face the challenge of fixing our food environment head on,' said Food Foundation executive director Anna Taylor.

'Bold action will be required if we are to safeguard the future health of our children – but is by no means impossible.'

The Food Foundation report, now in its third year, uses 10 different metrics to analyse and track the progress of the UK food system. This year's report was produced in collaboration with Nielsen, Eating Better, Action on Sugar and the University of Cambridge, among others.

7 July 2021

www.thegrocer.co.uk

Families have high awareness of healthy eating but low income means many struggle to access good food

Low-income families have a high awareness of healthy diets but can't afford good quality and nutritious food, new research show.

The University of York study, in partnership with N8Agrifood, showed that participants tried to eat as much fruit and vegetables as they could within financial constraints, avoiding processed food wherever possible. But there was widespread acknowledgement that processed food was often more accessible than healthy options because of its lower cost.

The researchers said that while the diets of low-income households have been subject to much scrutiny and debate, there is currently limited evidence in the UK on the diet quality and food practices of households reporting food insecurity and food bank use.

Diet

Dr Maddy Power, from the Department of Health Sciences, said: 'This research explores lived experiences of food insecurity, the notion of individual 'choice' and the underlying drivers of diet quality among low income families.

'The findings suggest that educational interventions are likely to be less effective in tackling food insecurity and poor nutrition among people living on a low income, as the people who took part in our study had good knowledge about healthy diets, but quite simply couldn't afford to buy what was needed to maintain a recommended healthy diet.'

Participants reported that access to healthy and fresh food was further constrained by geographic access. The availability of fresh and healthy food in local shops was perceived to be poor, but the cost of travelling to large supermarkets, where the quality and diversity of food may be better, was considered prohibitively expensive.

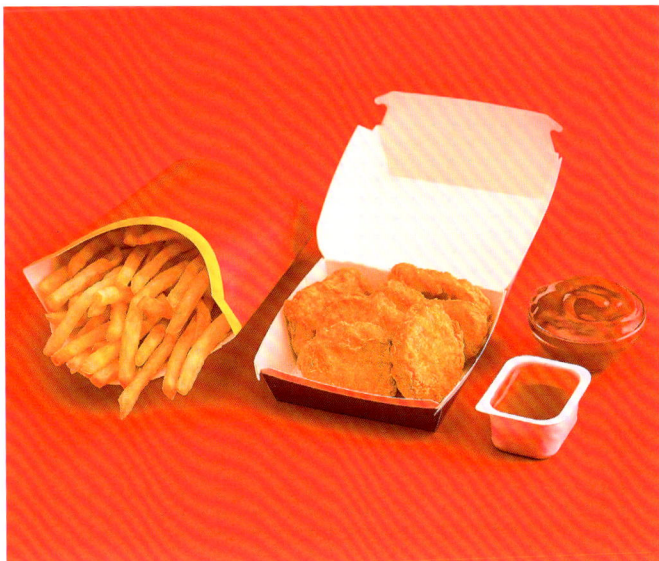

Stigma

Awareness of being priced out of nutritious and fresh food because of low income reinforced the stigma of living with poverty and was a very visible and everyday example of socio-economic inequality particularly for parents and caregivers, who were keen to ensure their children had access to a healthy diet.

One respondent said, 'It's not nice to feel you can't buy food that is healthy or better because it's more expensive.'

Other participants acknowledged that processed food was often more accessible than 'healthy' options because of its lower cost with one person saying: 'Healthy food is expensive and unhealthy food is cheap.'

Researchers say policies focusing on addressing structural drivers, including poverty and geographical access to food, are needed.

Food bank

The research also suggested a relationship between higher processed food consumption and having used a food bank.

Researchers say that the pandemic and the associated economic fallout has precipitated a sharp increase in food insecurity in the UK. In July 2020, roughly 16 per cent of adults – equivalent to 7.8 million people – reduced meal sizes or skipped meals due to insufficient income for food. This figure, which remained stable between April and July 2020, is roughly double rates of food insecurity before Covid-19.

The study took place between 2018 and 2020 and involved participatory research conducted with families of primary school age children.

Dr Katie Jayne Pybus and Professor Kate Pickett from the Department of Health Sciences and Professor Bob Doherty from The York Management School also contributed to the research.

About this research
The paper titled, *"The reality is that on Universal Credit I cannot provide the recommended amount of fresh fruit and vegetables per day for my children": Moving the conversation from a behavioural to a systemic understanding of food practices and purchases* is published in Emerald Open Research as part of the N8Agrifood Collection.

23 February 2021

Levelling up on local food environments

In the Serving Up Levelling Up blog series we'll be exploring how food and diets will need to be an essential part of the Government's levelling up agenda if it is going to achieve its ambition to level up the UK.

By Shona Goudie

In the *Levelling Up White Paper* published earlier this month, Government set out 12 missions to achieve their ambition to level up the country and ensure equal opportunity across the UK. Food and diets will need to be an essential part of the Government's levelling up agenda if it is going to achieve these missions. In this blog, we explore the role of food in the mission to boost local pride and how transforming local food environments should be part of revitalising and regenerating our high streets.

> **'By 2030, pride in place, such as people's satisfaction with their town centre and engagement in local culture and community, will have risen in every area of the UK, with the gap between top performing and other areas closing.'**
>
> *– Levelling Up White Paper*

Food environments (our surroundings that influence how we engage with the food system) are not supporting us to make healthy dietary choices, particularly in more deprived areas of the UK. The Food Foundation's *Broken Plate* demonstrates how difficult it is to eat healthily when there are so many factors such as affordability, availability, convenience and marketing making it easier to make the unhealthy choice even when we know this is bad for our health and the planet.

Our local town and city centres form part of this food environment: our high streets are filled with fast food takeaways and we are bombarded by outdoor advertising of unhealthy foods further influencing us to make unhealthy choices.

Advertising

Outdoor advertising surrounds us in our towns and cities - on public transport, on bus stops, on train stations, and on billboards. 98% of the UK population are exposed to outdoor advertising every day.[1] A study in the North East of England found that approximately 1 in 2 adverts on bus shelters were for food and non-alcoholic drinks and of these over a third were for less healthy products.[2] We know that advertising spend on food and non-alcoholic drink is disproportionately spent on unhealthy products,[3] and research shows that obesity rates are likely to be higher in areas with more outdoor advertising of unhealthy foods.[4]

Advertising of food can be used in a positive way to boost health. The Veg Power campaign has demonstrated that with their Eat Them To Defeat Them campaign finding that

advertising vegetables helped to increase consumption.[5] Current commitments to restrict advertising of food and drink which is high in fat, salt and/or sugar (HFSS) are focused on TV and online, but there is a significant gap by not banning this type of advertising in outdoor spaces.

Last week, the London School of Hygiene and Tropical Medicine published a study showing that polices to restrict advertising of unhealthy food are effective at helping to improve diets – they found that the ban on advertising HFSS food and drink on the Transport for London network was associated with households in London buying 1000 fewer calories of HFSS in their weekly shop and decreased calories from chocolate and sweets by 20%.[6]

The Grocer revealed last week that as many as 70 local authorities are planning to introduce similar policies following the success in London.[7] This shows that there is appetite for local government to make these changes to our local food environments.

Furthermore, people don't want to be bombarded by advertising of unhealthy foods – citizens said this clearly during the Public Dialogues for the National Food Strategy[8] and findings from research across the board shows the majority of people support bans on advertising of these products.[9, 10, 11]

> **'What advertisers will do as well is blame individuals for the choices we are making as do the government in a lot of their campaigns. It's like this is your choice, you're making the bad choice and you're choosing these things, but actually that's not what happens, it's not the individuals, it's the subliminal messaging and it's the food environment.'**
>
> *— Food Foundation Veg Advocate*

Fast food takeaways

It's not uncommon in the UK to see streets with wall-to-wall takeaways. One in four places to buy food are fast food outlets making these unhealthy foods the most convenient option for lots of people.[12] The density of fast-food outlets is much higher in the North than the South, and varies widely across local authorities in England – in the Isles of Scilly 6% of food outlets are fast food outlets but in Blackburn with Darwen it's as high as 39%.[13]

The Levelling Up White Paper reflects that 'economic and social disparities are often reflected in places' built environment' – this is the case with fast food takeaways. The density of fast-food outlets is greater in more deprived areas – almost as twice as high in the most deprived local authorities compared with the least deprived. Easier access to neighbourhood takeaway outlets has been shown to increase consumption of takeaways and is associated with higher weight.[14] Not only are takeaways damaging our health, they can create less pleasant neighbourhoods to be living in. Enforcing stricter regulations on fast food locations could simultaneously deliver benefits in tackling health disparities and increases people's satisfaction with the areas they live in.

I'm thinking of, the top of our street, there's maybe 3 or 4 takeaways and a Sainsbury's, but when I was growing up on the same parade there was a bakery, a greengrocers and a fish mongers, they've just all gone now they're just replaced with fried chicken and Indian, burger places'

– Food Foundation Veg Advocate

There are currently policies which give potential for local planners to regulate takeaways but there are a number of barriers to implementing them. Some areas do regulate, but 80% of takeaway food outlet planning criteria are not health-focused.[15]

Last week, South Tyneside Council refused plans for new food takeaways saying this would clash with their policies to promote healthy lifestyles and tackle obesity.[16] This shows that it is possible for local areas to do more to regulate fast food takeaways and improve food environments.

Conclusion

Creating a healthier local food environment has potential to deliver on levelling up both on health and local pride. As part of the effort to empower local leadership, councils and local authorities need to be better supported and encouraged to use the powers available to them to transform their town centres and high streets to facilitate better diets and health.

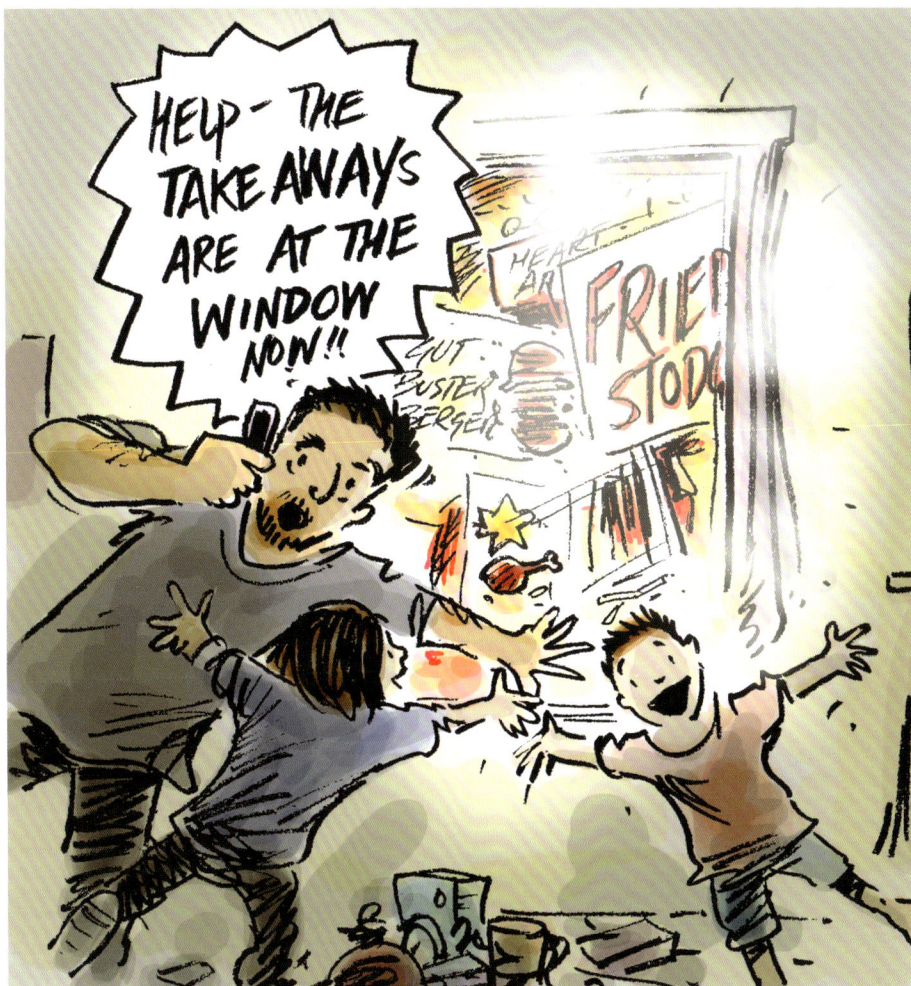

References

1. https://pubmed.ncbi.nlm.nih.gov/34974851/#:~:text=The%20 deprivation%20level%20of%20the,UK%20Index%20of%20Multiple%20 Deprivation.&text=Results%3A%20832%20advertisements%20were%20 identified,%2C%2035.1%25%20were%20less%20healthy.
2. https://pubmed.ncbi.nlm.nih.gov/34974851/#:~:text=The%20 deprivation%20level%20of%20the,UK%20Index%20of%20Multiple%20 Deprivation.&text=Results%3A%20832%20advertisements%20were%20 identified,%2C%2035.1%25%20were%20less%20healthy.
3. https://foodfoundation.org.uk/publication/broken-plate-2021
4. https://www.sustainweb.org/publications/feb22-advertising-policy-toolkit/
5. https://ifour-vegpower-uploads.s3.eu-west-2.amazonaws.com/wp-content/uploads/2021/10/07180045/Eat-Them-to-Defeat-Them-2021-Concise-Report-.pdf
6. https://journals.plos.org/plosmedicine/article?id=10.1371/journal.pmed.1003915
7. https://www.thegrocer.co.uk/health/councils-set-to-follow-tfl-in-junk-food-ad-crackdown/664626.article
8. https://www.nationalfoodstrategy.org/wp-content/uploads/2021/09/HVM-National-Food-Strategy-Public-Dialogue-report-Sep21.pdf
9. https://yougov.co.uk/topics/food/articles-reports/2021/06/07/advertising-ban-on-junk-food-poll
10. https://www.ipsos.com/en-uk/public-supports-government-intervention-diet-health-and-advertising
11. https://www.health.org.uk/publications/reports/public-perceptions-of-health-and-social-care-in-light-of-covid-19-may-2020
12. https://foodfoundation.org.uk/publication/broken-plate-2021
13. https://foodfoundation.org.uk/publication/broken-plate-2021
14. https://researchonline.lshtm.ac.uk/id/eprint/4655475/
15. https://reader.elsevier.com/reader/sd/pii/S1353829218310414?token
16. https://www.bbc.co.uk/news/uk-england-tyne-60359720

23 February 2022

www.foodfoundation.org.uk

How to navigate healthy eating with kids without triggering problems down the line

Parents are always looking for ways for their children to stay happy and healthy – and food is a huge part of this.

By Lizzie Thomson

Parents are always looking for ways for their children to stay happy and healthy – and food is a huge part of this.

It's a topic that's more relevant than ever, too – with the pandemic contributing to soaring rates of childhood obesity, type 2 diabetes and blood pressure, mostly linked to an increase in takeaways and super-processed foods.

But talking to children about food requires a delicate balancing act. After all, even well- meaning comments can have a knock-on effect on a child's long-term relationship with food.

So how can parents navigate healthy eating without promoting problems down the line?

Ultimately, it's all about fostering healthy eating habits – without encouraging disordered eating or food shaming.

Experts have shared some ways to approach healthy eating with kids, as well as some key things to avoid.

Focus on health, rather than weight

Psychologist Dr. Amanda Gummer, founder of The Good Play Guide, explains that it's all about focusing on the health benefits to healthy eating, rather than weight.

She says: 'The focus when talking about healthy eating should be on growing a healthy body, rather than looking a certain way.

'It's likely they'll be learning about this in school, so start by finding out what they know already, and build on this.

'Talk about all of the things your body needs to be healthy, and how a balanced diet contributes to this.'

Don't ban foods – or label things as 'good' or 'bad'

Banning certain foods, like junk food, fuels the idea that some foods are 'bad' and some are 'good' – which can lead to a dangerous relationship with food.

'It's important to teach children how to eat foods like this in moderation,' explains Amanda.

'At some point your child will go out on their own and be responsible for their own diet.

'By banning a particular type of food, there's a risk that they will just binge on this as soon as they are able to, because they haven't learned how to manage this. Keep in mind that this does not include energy drinks, which are not appropriate for those under 16.

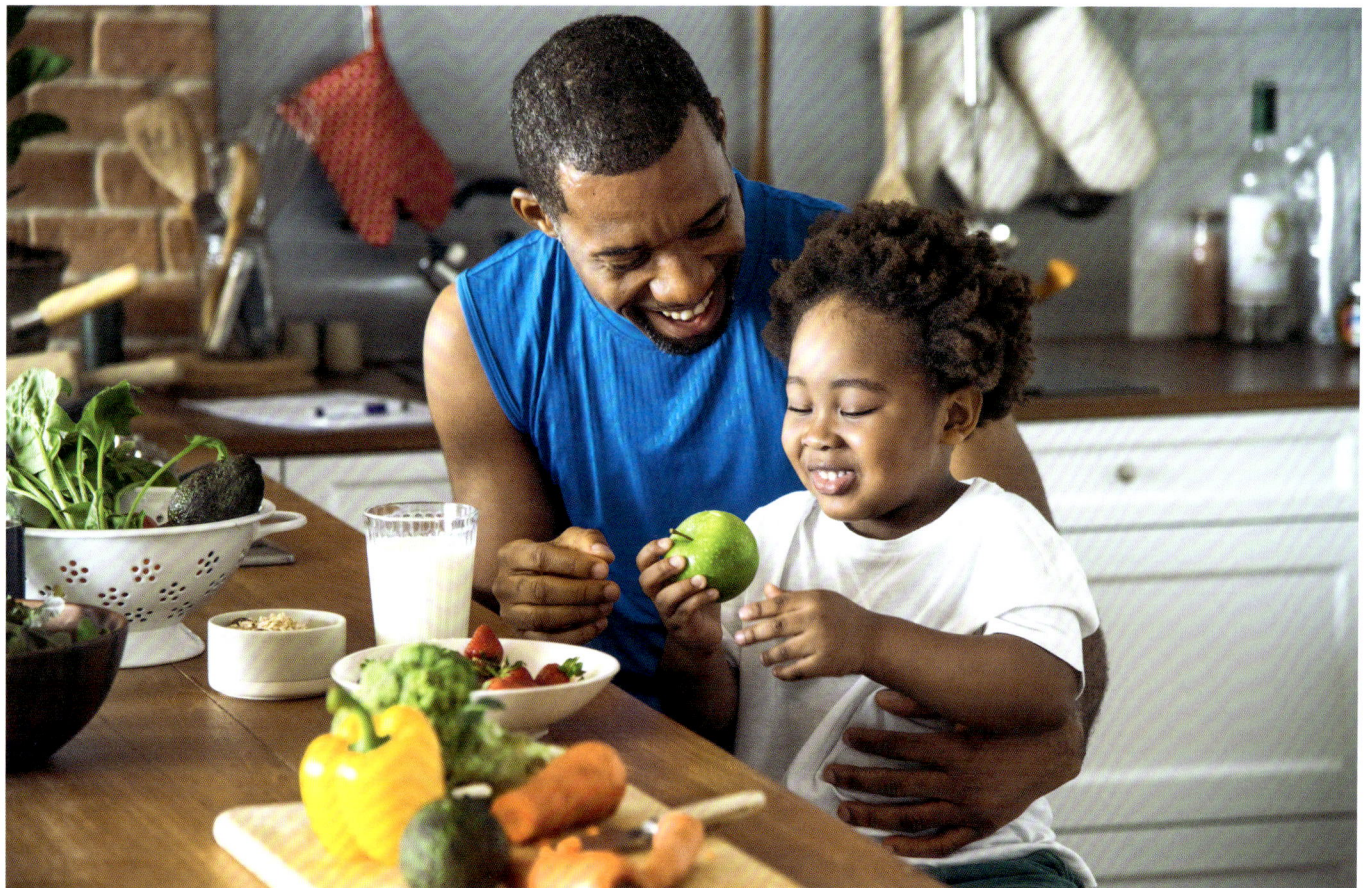

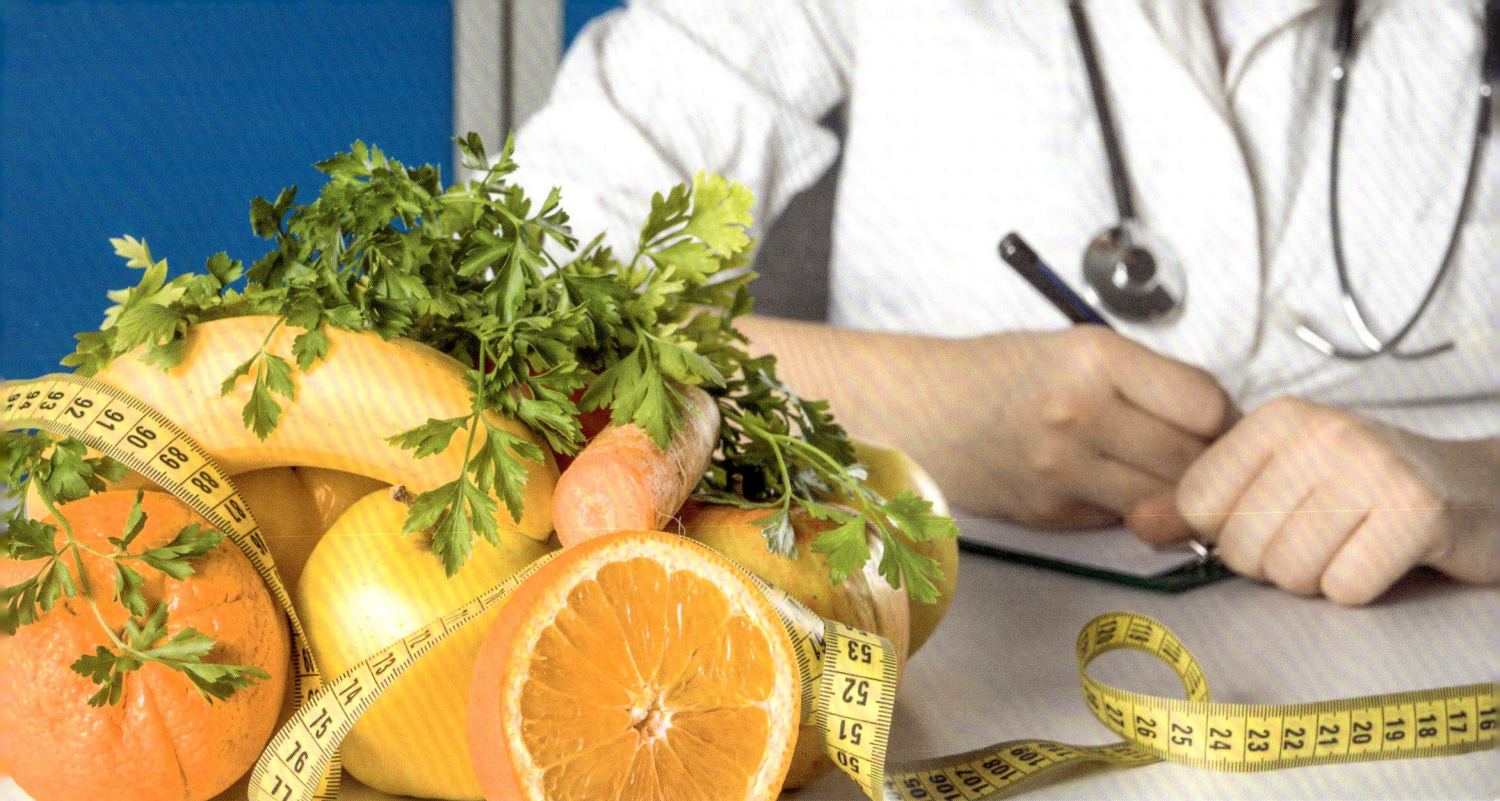

'In this instance, I would discuss it with your child and help them understand why energy drinks are not recommended for them.'

Try not to use junk as a reward

Giving a child junk food as a reward also plays into this narrative.

'It's also a good idea to avoid using junk food, such as sweets, as a reward,' continues Amanda. 'Instead, use things such as time at the playground, a movie night, or craft activity as rewards.

'This is so your child doesn't see junk food as "good" and healthy food as "bad."'

Model positive body image

We all know young children are like sponges, they soak up the information and attitudes of the people around them.

As a result, it's important to champion positive attitudes to food and a confident body image – so your child can copy you.

'For example, avoid talking about how you wish you were thinner, or more muscly, less wrinkly or saggy in front of them. Instead, try to love your body the way it is and be outspoken about this,' adds Amanda.

'By doing this, you may encourage your child to look for the things they like about themselves too, and respect that everyone looks different.'

Don't lecture

Studies have shown that parenting lectures are not only boring but ineffective, too

Dr Lynne Green, the chief clinical officer at Kooth, says: 'Don't lecture your child on what they should and shouldn't be eating – this can create resentment and disengagement.'

Instead, try and get kids involved and interested in a fun way – this could be asking them to help you with the food shop or meal planning healthy dinner options together.

Listen to concerns and be honest with answers

'If your children asks about being thin or fat, or eating disorders, have an age-appropriate conversation with them,' adds Amanda.

'If they are asking these questions they deserve an honest, considered answer.

'One way you can make sure your answers are age-appropriate is to clarify what the question is, to make sure you are giving them the information they are looking for.'

Lynne adds that it's also important to listen to your child's point of view and validate how they might be feeling – even if you might be struggling to make sense of it yourself.

Know when it's time to seek professional help

'For those who are concerned about a child with a very low calorie intake, worried about making things worse by confronting the issue or find themselves thinking "at least they are eating something which is better than nothing at all," I would urge you to seek professional help,' says Lynne.

'Similarly, if you feel your child is overeating and struggling to maintain a healthy body mass index (a better measure than weight alone), reach out for help.

'Put simply, a child who is not well nourished is at greater risk of developing a range of emotional, physical, and social difficulties.'

17 March 2022

What is the National Food Strategy and how could it change the way England eats?

An article from *The Conversation*.

By Kelly Parsons, Food Systems Policy & Governance Research Fellow, University of Hertfordshire & David Barling, Professor of Food Policy and Security, Director of the Centre for Agriculture, Food and Environmental Management, University of Hertfordshire

THE CONVERSATION

Reforming England's food system could save the country £126 billion, according to a recent government-commissioned report. *The National Food Strategy*, led by British businessman Henry Dimbleby, proposes a raft of measures to shake up how food is produced and the kinds of diets most people eat.

The need for action is laid out in stark terms. Poor diets contribute to around 64,000 deaths every year in England, and the government spends £18 billion a year treating obesity-related conditions. How we grow food accounts for a quarter of greenhouse gas emissions and is the leading cause of biodiversity destruction.

To meet these challenges, the report calls for 'escaping the junk food cycle' to improve general health and reduce the strain on the NHS, reducing the gap in good diets between high- and low-income areas, using space more efficiently to grow food so that more land can return to nature, and creating a long-term shift in food culture.

The strategy is, in parts, highly ambitious, particularly in its framing of the challenge as a systemic issue, and in some of the more innovative measures it proposes.

These include the world's first sugar and salt reformulation tax, aimed at forcing manufacturers to make the foods they sell healthier – by reformulating recipes to remove sugar and salt – and raising around £3 billion for the Treasury in the process. Companies would also have to report how healthy and sustainable their food sales are. Cannily, the strategy team persuaded some companies to come out in favour of the proposals, which suggests they're serious about seeing their ideas implemented and attuned to the government's nervousness around upsetting the food industry.

The Eatwell Guide, which shows what proportion of our diet should come from each food group, would be based not only on the healthiness of certain foods, but their environmental sustainability too. This reference diet would underpin government decisions, and help ensure food policies are consistent with what is good for people and the planet.

The strategy takes a commendably bold stance on the government's approach to trade policy, making clear that not honouring a manifesto commitment to protect food standards could bankrupt Britain's farming sector.

Missed opportunities

At the same time, the strategy is politically pragmatic, clearly crafted with an eye on what is likely to be winnable within the current government. As such, some politically-contentious issues are sidestepped.

The strategy sets a goal of reducing meat consumption by 30% over ten years, but shies away from interventions to tackle this head on, with a meat tax discounted as 'politically impossible'.

The report notably fails to address the poorly paid, precarious and often dangerous jobs of food workers, in agriculture and hospitality. The report details how the problems with food are systemic, but misses the chance to make the link between poor working conditions in the sector and food insecurity and health. The terrible irony of 'critical workers' like farmers, fishers and catering staff that feed many of us is that they're unable to afford to eat well themselves.

The scale of the challenge has led to calls for a new minister for hunger, a cabinet sub-committee on food, or an independent food body. The strategy opts instead for a Good Food Bill with statutory targets around diet-related health and reporting. It also favours expanding the remit of the Food Standards Agency (FSA) to encompass health and sustainability and calls for improved monitoring and measurement of the food system and the policies linked to it.

If enacted, these proposals could benefit food policymaking, but they'd leave the difficult question of how different government departments can coordinate on the issue untouched. Expanding an existing body may be politically expedient, but does the non-ministerial FSA have the clout and capacity to drive reform in the many other departments with a hand in food policy?

An ambitious and innovate strategy in parts, and wise for its political astuteness. Whether it has achieved the right balance will become clearer in the next phase, when the Department for Environment, Food & Rural Affairs delivers its response. The recommendations will need to survive the political jungle and overcome obstacles both bureaucratic and ideological.

Should they make it through in one piece, these policies could tackle some of the biggest challenges related to food. But more importantly, the strategy could disrupt the politics and ideas about what people should want from their food system, and give licence to additional policy interventions in trade, meat and jobs.

21 July 2021

Food retailers' promotional strategies – a missed opportunity to improve people's health

This Salt Awareness Week, we look at how food retailers shape our daily salt intake and its negative health impacts through promotion of unhealthy foods – and how investors can act collaboratively to make them create better food environments.

By Elinor George, Project and Impact Manager - Health, ShareAction

A healthy diet is a key building block in contributing to an individual's health.

But an individual's diet is heavily influenced by wider determinants including the environment in which they find themselves, and the products that companies promote.

Each year, Action on Salt organises a national "Salt Awareness Week" to raise awareness of the effect of too much salt on our health.

This week (14th-20th March 2022) they have been shining a light on the salt content of our favourite food products, particularly those included in high street store meal deal combos.

Adults should eat no more than 6g of salt per day, but the average person in the UK is thought to eat around 8g per day (PHE, 2016). Too much salt in someone's diet can raise blood pressure, increasing the risk of heart disease and stroke.

Retailers contribute hugely to our daily salt intake

Action on Salt's recent report on the nutritional value of meal deal combos at eight high street stores found that:

◆ Almost three quarters of snacks included in these deals are dangerously high in saturated fat, salt and sugar (HFSS). The worst offender, Co-op Lemon and Coriander Green Olives, has 2.02g salt per pack – almost a third of overall daily intake.

◆ Nearly one in three snacks in these deals exceed their maximum salt target, including Ginsters Cornish Pasty 180g (1.89g of salt, more salt than 5.5 packets of ready salted crisps) and Jacob's mini cheddars 50g (1.2g of salt, more salt than 3 Mini Babybel)

Around one in three people buy a meal deal at least twice a week. This daily promotion of products high in salt across retailers is therefore having a hugely negative impact on people's health.

Retailers have a big influence over the food available to us

These findings show that manufacturers and retailers need to do more to support better diets.

In spite of voluntary government salt reduction targets, manufacturers and retailers are continuing to flood the market with unhealthy products.

Some retailers are performing better than others: Sainsbury's snacks rank more favourably. According to Action on Salt's report, Sainsbury's offers a higher proportion of non-HFSS snacks, which are closer to the regulation targets. Meanwhile, Asda and Subway have the highest proportion (82 per cent) of HFSS snacks in their meal deals.

In December 2021, we shared similar findings from the research foundation Questionmark. It tracked all promotions of food products in the four biggest supermarkets – Asda, Morrisons, Sainsbury's and Tesco.

The research found that up to 43 per cent of the promotions held across the stores over a five week period were for unhealthy products, and 50 per cent of meal deal product promotions were high in fat, salt or sugar.

This shows that companies are missing out on an opportunity to support better health and stay clear of possible further regulations in this space.

Investors have the power to change our food environment

We need to create healthier food environments for the UK's physical and economic health.

According to Public Health England, a reduction in average salt intake from 8g to 6g per day is estimated to prevent over 8000 premature deaths each year and save the NHS over £570 million annually.

Through our Healthy Markets initiative and investor coalition, we influence manufacturers, such as Unilever, and retailers, such as Tesco, to encourage these companies to increase their reporting and set targets on their proportion of sales from healthy products.

Given that UK consumers spent £96 billion on food and non-alcoholic drinks in the grocery sector, if retailers were to prioritise and promote healthy products, they could have a huge impact on the nation's diet.

Investors have the power to change to shape our food environments for the better, and the Healthy Markets Initiative is the way to make it a reality.

18 March 2022

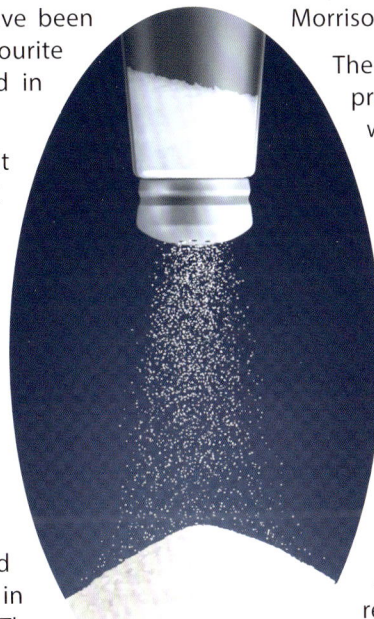

What is the future of appetite and obesity research?

Widespread problems of obesity, food insecurity and diet-related ill health require a dramatic change in our food environment, but how can research help to tackle these issues?

By Dr Aaron Lett – Imperial College London, Dr Chris McLeod – Loughborough University, Dr Sarah Sauchell – University of Bristol and Dr Sion Parry – University of Oxford

Food reformulation and innovation to influence healthy and sustainable diets

Food reformulation is a route to providing foods that may be lower in energy and nutrients we should be eating less of (e.g. saturated fats, sugars and salt) but that can still be convenient, appealing and affordable. Effective reformulation, however, is more complex than simply removing or reducing such target nutrients from food and drink products. There are significant barriers including ingredient and food-specific technical challenges that need to be overcome without adversely impacting shelf life and sensory appeal or indeed having potentially unintended adverse health effects: for example, if reducing the sugars content is compensated for by an increase in saturated fat.

The popular demand for 'clean label' also offers a reformulation challenge for businesses, with consumers looking for few ingredients, that they perceive as 'natural' and avoiding ingredients such as low calorie sweeteners. Furthermore, consumer demand, corporate responsibility or government pressure may all be instrumental in incentivising food manufacturers to reformulate products.

Versatile multifunctional ingredients, innovative strategies that encourage long term repeat purchases, as well as insights into consumer purchasing behaviour are needed to help ensure that reformulated foods have a positive health impact and are commercially viable. Fundamentally such foods need to be designed around, and validated to improve human health.

Use of 'Big data' to develop understanding of drivers of appetite and food choice

'Big data' refers to large datasets which can be analysed to identify patterns and trends in complex behaviours (e.g. data from smartphones, wearable devices and social media). Although in obesity research big data can help to better understand drivers of appetite and food choice, to date its potential remains largely untapped.

To harness the true functionality of big data, we need to reduce the risk of collecting imprecise or inaccurate data and prevent the potential of flawed information being used in the implementation of interventions and policies. Smartphones and wearable devices offer great potential for collecting big data, but this method may only tap into more affluent sectors, so the results may not be generalisable to lower socioeconomic status population groups. Long term relationships need to be established with companies (e.g. supermarkets) that have access to big data e.g. scanned consumer purchase data, with the challenges of obtaining permission to use such company data for research purposes overcome. Finally, research will need to integrate a wide range of data; from small studies examining individual food choice behaviour or hormone secretion, to larger datasets examining social contributors to obesity (e.g. increased prevalence of fast food availability).

Big data may be 'the future' in many research fields. However, in appetite and obesity research, further groundwork is needed to ensure that findings are beneficial, timely, do not exacerbate inequalities and are ethically sound.

One diet does not fit all – bridging the gap between appetite research and obesity services

Whilst food reformulation and big data can help tackle obesity and gain insight on a larger scale, we must also acknowledge individual variability in responses to weight management interventions and the need for interindividual differences to be reflected in quality obesity services.

To guide personalised care we need to improve collaboration between researchers and healthcare teams. Novel insights into appetite regulation generated from big data, clinical research and patient experience can be used within healthcare teams to individualise treatment plans. We should also aim for an integrated model of care where every patient in a wide range of clinics can be a research participant, with better coordinated UK-wide trial systems that facilitate approval, recruitment, data collection and access to data sets. NHS commissioners could play a key role in helping researchers trial novel interventions within existing care protocols, and in finding ways to make data collected in clinics readily available for research. They can also reinforce the importance of evaluating quality of life and overall health, which are essential for long term weight management.

Low income areas lack of healthy options

Cravings for sugars and saturated fat

Ads targeting children's eating habits

Too many diet options?

Is this healthy for me?

Am I obese?

Eating habits

Promoting healthy options

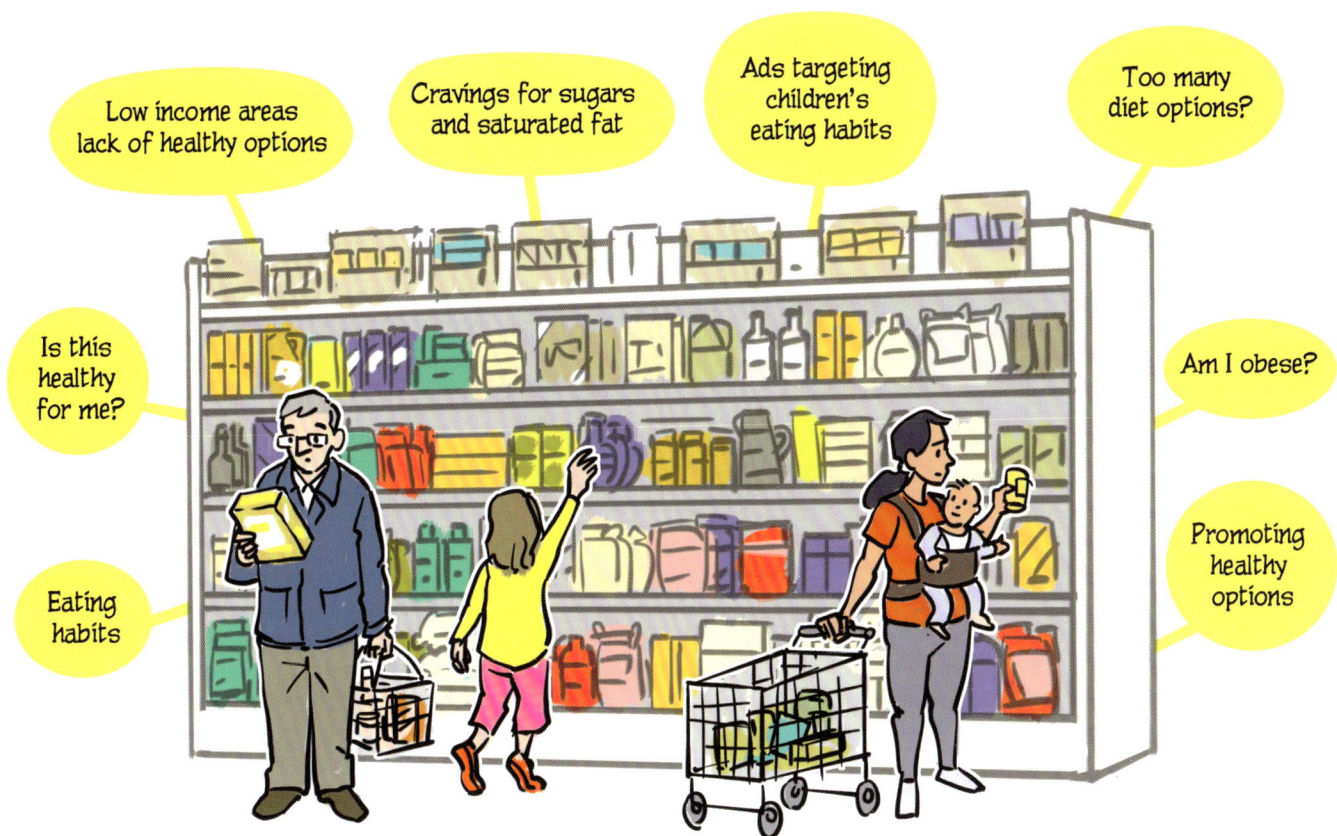

Having systems that allow an understanding of what is effective for patients with similar profiles including genetic composition, endocrine function (e.g. insulin resistance), psychological barriers to behaviour change (e.g. vulnerability to external stressors) and immediate social environment will open doors to personalising obesity treatment.

Supporting behaviour change - environmental drivers of obesity and food choices

Overall, we should move towards a 'whole systems approach,' which aims to integrate all the various stakeholders within a system (e.g. patients, public health workers, local businesses etc.) to collectively tackle obesity. For this kind of strategy to be successful, infrastructure and resources must be in place across the UK. This may include lifestyle weight management programmes, appropriately trained healthcare professionals who are aware of, and can make referrals to, weight management programmes, community groups that can offer additional peer support, and more widespread restrictions around food advertising.

The challenges of adopting this approach are numerous. Some local authorities, for instance, use quicker, more simple 'sticking plaster'-type solutions; an example of which can be seen for the nation's other nutrition crisis, food poverty, where food banks are the preferred management strategy rather than addressing underlying causes. Developing tools to measure system changes may help overcome some of these barriers. Demonstrating that we can accurately monitor how new strategies involving multiple stakeholders impact behaviour and how this may help to tackle obesity will provide evidence of the potential benefits of using this approach for local governments and funders. We must also investigate ways to effectively engage stakeholders (e.g. via social networking sites) to ensure inclusivity.

Cross-discipline, collaborative research is key to driving change in this area.

2021

Key Facts

- Energy intake (calories) should be in balance with energy expenditure. To avoid unhealthy weight gain, total fat should not exceed 30% of total energy intake. (page 1)

- Limiting intake of free sugars to less than 10% of total energy intake is part of a healthy diet. (page 1)

- Keeping salt intake to less than 5g per day helps to prevent hypertension, and reduces the risk of heart disease and stroke in the adult population. (page 1)

- Eating at least 400g, or five portions, of fruit and vegetables per day reduces the risk of NCDs and helps to ensure an adequate daily intake of dietary fibre. (page 2)

- In May 2014 WHO set up the Commission on Ending Childhood Obesity. In 2016, the Commission proposed a set of recommendations to successfully tackle childhood and adolescent obesity in different contexts around the world. (page 4).

- We can go for 50 days without food, but only two to three without water. Water is essential to the human body and we need about 2.5 litres of water a day. (page 5)

- Eating too much sugar is a major cause of tooth decay and excess weight. While sugar consumption remains too high, since 2008 there has been a steady decline in sugar intake in both children and adults. (page 8)

- There has been a fall in red and processed meat consumption over the past decade, most likely for environmental and health reasons. Significantly, all adults now consume, on average, below the maximum recommended daily intake of red and processed meat (70g per day). (page 8)

- WHO recommends that less than 30% of our energy intake comes from fats, and that unsaturated fats found in vegetable oils (such as olive, sunflower, canola and soybean oils) are preferable to saturated fats from animal products such as butter, cream, cheese, ghee and lard. (page 11)

- According to a 2020 survey by the European Consumer Organisation (BEUC), foods that are 'minimal processed, traditional' matter to consumers. Such foods are most valued by consumers in Portugal, Greece and Lithuania, who associate them with 'sustainable food'. (page 16)

- In Europe, the food industry employs close to 5 million people and boasts a turnover of €1.2 trillion, which would be significantly impacted without the processing of food and food ingredients. (page 17)

- Foods are divided into four categories – unprocessed or minimally processed, culinary ingredients, processed, and ultra-processed – according to the way the food is used and how much it has been tinkered with during production. (page 19)

- National advice on how much red meat people should eat regularly varies, ranging from a maximum recommended intake of 70g a day (350g per week) in the UK to 500g a week in Scandinavian countries. (page 21)

- In the UK, it is estimated that 3.8 million people aged over 16 years have been diagnosed with diabetes and nearly 1 million are unaware that they have the condition. (page 22)

- About 90% of people with diabetes have type 2 diabetes. (page 22)

- Although obesity has risen for all ages, the most worrying age group is those within their last year of primary school. Here, general rates have risen from 21% to 25%. However, in poorer areas, rates have increased by twice the amount. (page 25)

- The annual *Broken Plate report* found that the average cost of healthy food in 2019 was around £7.68. This is much higher than the £2.48 cost of less healthy food with the same caloric intake. (page 25)

- According to the *Broken Plate report*, foods that are high in sugar and fat are only 40% of the cost of fruit & vegetables per each 1,000 calories. (page 30)

- The poorest fifth of the country's households would need to spend 40% of their income on healthier food to be able to meet the government's Eatwell Guide costs, compared with 5% for the wealthiest fifth. (page 30)

- A study in the North East of England found that approximately 1 in 2 adverts on bus shelters were for food and non-alcoholic drinks and of these over a third were for less healthy products. (page 32)

- The density of fast-food outlets is much higher in the North than the South, and varies widely across local authorities in England – in the Isles of Scilly 6% of food outlets are fast food outlets but in Blackburn with Darwen it's as high as 39% (page 32)

- Poor diets contribute to around 64,000 deaths every year in England, and the government spends £18 billion a year treating obesity-related conditions. (page 36)

- According to Public Health England, a reduction in average salt intake from 8g to 6g per day is estimated to prevent over 8000 premature deaths each year and save the NHS over £570 million annually. (page 37)

Additives

Additives are ingredients used in the preparation of processed foods. Some of these are extracted from naturally occurring materials, others are manufactured chemicals. They may be added to food to stop it going bad (preservatives), improve its appearance (for example by changing its colour) or to enhance its flavour. Other types of additives include thickeners, sweeteners, emulsifiers and anti-caking agents, and there are many more.

BMI (body mass index)

An abbreviation which stands for 'body mass index' and is used to determine whether an individual's weight is in proportion to their height. If a person's BMI is below 18.5 they are usually seen as underweight. If a person has a BMI greater than or equal to 25, they are classed as overweight and a BMI of 30 and over is obese. As BMI is the same for both sexes and adults of all ages, it provides the most useful population-level measure of overweight and obesity. However, it should be considered a rough guide because it may not correspond to the same degree of 'fatness' in different individuals (e.g. a body builder could have a BMI of 30 but would not be obese because their weight would be primarily muscle rather than fat.

Diabetes (type 1 and type 2)

The main difference between the two types of diabetes is that type 1 diabetes is a genetic disorder that often shows up early in life, and type 2 is largely diet-related and develops over time.

Diet

The variety of foods and drink that someone consumes on a regular basis. The phrase 'on a diet' is also often used to refer to a period of controlling what one eats while trying to lose weight.

Dietary inequality

Where inequalities in the food system mean people in low-income groups eat less healthily than those on higher incomes.

Eatwell Guide

The Eatwell Guide has replaced the Eatwell plate. It shows the different types of food we need to eat – and in what proportions – to have a well-balanced and healthy diet. Based on the eatwell guide, people should try to eat: plenty of fruit and vegetables; plenty of potatoes, bread, rice, pasta and other starchy foods; some milk and dairy foods; some meat, fish, eggs, beans and other non-dairy sources of protein; and just a small amount of foods and drinks that are high in fat or sugar.

Food poverty

When people struggle to afford food. The UK has seen an increase in the use of food banks and food parcels. In 2020 approximately 2.5 million people used a food bank in the UK.

HFSS

HFSS stands for High in saturated Fat, Salt and Sugar. It is a description attributed to certain foods.

Junk food

'Junk' food is a widely used term for unhealthy and fatty foods with little nutritional value. It is usually associated with 'fast' or takeaway food.

National Food Strategy

The National Food Strategy was introduced in England in 2020. It's intention is to ensure that the food system delivers, safe, healthy, affordable food regardless of where people live or what they earn.

Nutrigenomics

Nutrigenomics (also known as nutritional genomics) is broadly defined as the relationship between nutrients, diet, and gene expression

Nutrition

The provision of materials needed by the body for growth, maintenance and sustaining life. Commonly when people talk about nutrition, they are referring to the healthy and balanced diet we all need to eat in order for the body to function properly.

Obesity

When someone is overweight to the extent that their BMI is 30 or above, they are classed as obese. Obesity is increasing in the UK and is associated with a number of health problems such as an increased risk of heart disease and type 2 diabetes. Worldwide obesity has more than doubled since 1980 and this is most likely due to our more sedentary lifestyle combined with a lack of physical exercise.

UPFS

UPFS stands for ultra-processed foods. These are foods that go through multiple processes, contain many additives. They are generally energy-dense, high in unhealthy types of fat, refined starches, free sugars and salt, and poor sources of fibre.

Activities

Brainstorming

♦ In small groups discuss what you know about healthy eating. Consider the following:

  · Why is a healthy diet important?

  · What is meant by dietary inequality?

  · What are the health risks of a poor diet?

♦ As a class, brainstorm factors that you think shape a person's diet. How many of these factors are external influences and how many are down to personal preferences?

♦ What are HFSS foods?

♦ What is BMI?

Research

♦ In pairs, make a list of the health pros and cons of one of the following lifestyle diets:

  · Vegetarian

  · Vegan

  · Flexitarian.

♦ Over the course of a week, keep a record of how many portions of fruit and veg you eat in a day. Have you eaten more or less than you thought? Compare your findings with the rest of your class.

♦ Over the course of one day, if available, collect and read the nutritional information on any meals and snacks you eat. Add up the total amount of salt and sugar you have consumed that day. Is it under or over the RDI? Are you surprised by your results?

♦ Take a look at a TV guide and make a note of how many cookery and food-related programmes are shown across the five main channels in a week. In small groups, discuss if you have watched any of the shows before, and which, if any, emphasised nutrition and healthy eating.

♦ Choose a country in Europe and research their relationship with food. How healthy are their traditional dishes compared to the UK?

♦ Take a trip into your nearest town or city centre. Make a note of how many advertisements you see for fast food/soft drinks on billboards or on public transport. How many fast food outlets can you spot in the area?

Design

♦ Create a poster for your school or college canteen promoting healthy eating and highlighting the healthiest options on the menu.

♦ Choose one of the articles from this book and create your own illustration that depicts the key themes/messages from that article.

♦ Design an informative leaflet about the importance of vitamins and minerals in your diet.

♦ Create a social media campaign encouraging people to cut down their sugar consumption.

Oral

♦ In pairs, discuss whether you think you can eat a healthy balanced diet without consuming animal products.

♦ In small groups, talk about what 'dietary inequality' means and the reasons you think it exists in the UK.

♦ Choose one of the illustrations from this book and, with a partner, discuss what you think the artist was trying to portray.

♦ In pairs role play a situation in which one of you is a vegetarian trying to persuade your omnivore friend to eat less meat.

Reading/writing

♦ Write a menu plan for breakfast, lunch, evening meal and snacks for someone at risk of developing Type 2 diabetes. Use the information provided on page 24 for guidance about the best foods to include.

♦ Write a letter to your head teacher explaining why you believe it is important for students to be taught about diet and nutrition in school.

♦ Read the article *The alarming truth about ultra-processed foods and why you should stop eating them* (page 19). Write a list of examples of foods that belong in the following categories:

  · Unprocessed or minimally processed foods

  · Processed culinary ingredients

  · Processed foods

  · Ultra-processed foods

♦ Read the article *What is the National Food Strategy and how could it change the way England eats?* (page 36) and write a short paragraph summarising the objectives of the National Food Strategy.

Acknowledgements

The publisher is grateful for permission to reproduce the material in this book. While every care has been taken to trace and acknowledge copyright, the publisher tenders its apology for any accidental infringement or where copyright has proved untraceable. The publisher would be pleased to come to a suitable arrangement in any such case with the rightful owner.

The material reproduced in **issues** books is provided as an educational resource only. The views, opinions and information contained within reprinted material in **issues** books do not necessarily represent those of Independence Educational Publishers and its employees.

Images

Cover image courtesy of iStock. All other images courtesy Freepik, Pixabay & Unsplash.

Illustrations

Simon Kneebone: pages 2, 17 & 33. Angelo Madrid: pages 9,26 &39

Additional acknowledgements

Page 1 - Healthy diet: https://www.who.int/news-room/fact-sheets/detail/healthy-diet

With thanks to the Independence team: Shelley Baldry, Klaudia Sommer and Jackie Staines. Contributing Editor: Tracy Biram

Danielle Lobban

Cambridge, June 2022